The Pill

John Guillebaud is a consultant gynaecologist at the Hospital for Women in Soho Square, London, and Medical Director of the Margaret Pyke Centre. The Centre was opened by the Duke of Edinburgh in 1969, as a memorial to one of the pioneers of the family planning movement in Britain. It is within the National Health Service, and with about 45,000 annual attendances it is now the largest fertility centre in Europe. Couples are helped either to avoid an unplanned pregnancy or to overcome some difficulty in starting a family. Hundreds of medical students, doctors, and nurses are trained each year at the Centre, and new methods of birth control are investigated with the help of the Margaret Pyke Memorial Trust.

Dr Guillebaud was born in Burundi, Africa, and educated in Kenya and Britain. Soon after qualifying in medicine from Cambridge he spent six months as Medical Officer on the Royal Society Expedition to Mato Grosso, Brazil (1967–1968). He has travelled to every continent promoting planned parenthood and concern for the environment. He is a member of several expert committees, including the Advisory Committee on Contraception of the Medical Research Council. His wife Gwyneth is a family planning nurse, and they have three young children.

John Guillebaud

The Pill

Third Edition

OXFORD UNIVERSITY PRESS

1984

Oxford University Press, Walton Street, Oxford OX2 6DP

London New York Toronto
Delhi Bombay Calcutta Madras Karachi
Kuala Lumpur Singapore Hong Kong Tokyo
Nairobi Dar es Salaam Cape Town
Melbourne Auckland

and associated companies in
Beirut Berlin Ibadan Mexico City Nicosia

First published 1980
Second Edition 1983
Third Edition 1984

British Library Cataloguing in Publication Data
Guillebaud, John
The pill.—3rd ed.—(Oxford Paperbacks)
1. Oral contraceptives
1. Title
613.9'432 RG137.5
ISBN 0–19–286054–2

Library of Congress Cataloging in Publication Data
Guillebaud, John.
The pill.
Bibliography: p.
Includes index.
1. Oral contraceptives. I. Title. [DNLM: 1. Contra-
ceptives, Oral—popular works. QV 177 G958p]
RG137.5.G84 1984 613.9'432 84–9689
ISBN 0–19–286054–2

Printed in Great Britain by
Hazell Watson & Viney Ltd.,
Aylesbury, Bucks.

Preface
to the third edition

Only four years have passed since the first edition. This implies not only that the book is meeting a real need, but also that there continue to be many new developments. The completely rewritten sections include those on cancer, long-term effects of the pill, and 'which pill should be chosen?' (pages 119–24, 126–30, and 171–80). These and a number of smaller, updating changes have been made in the light of the very latest information available in 1984. They are intended to preserve the position of this book as, so far as I know, the most up-to-date and comprehensive handbook on hormonal contraception available anywhere; which in turn explains why it is found on the bookshelves of so many doctors and nurses.

The book could not have been written without the help of many individuals. For reading part or all of the text and making suggestions I am grateful to the following, who are all experts of one kind or another – as researchers, providers, or consumers of the pill: Terry Baker, David Barlow, Toni Belfield, Mary Bollam, Walli Bounds, Peter Bowen-Simpkins, Althea Coates, Heather and Dany Goodman, Meg Goodman, Kathleen Hunt-ington, Clifford Kay, Barbara Law, Audrey Leathard, Jim Mann, Eric McGraw, Alexandra Monks, George Morris, John Newton, Zandria Pauncefort, Walter Prendiville, Maria Pursey, Jan Savage, Pram Senanayake, Susan Sleigh, Gordon Stirrat, and Martin Vessey.

Their comments were supplemented by those of my band of typists, whose patience in typing and retyping drafts was much appreciated: Diana Ager, Margaret Bailón, Eileen Farr, Jeanette Highsted, Irene Jeffery, Julia Kingston-Lee, Nanette Paine, Maxine Stone.

Helpful telephone assistance was provided by Peter Adams, Mark Belsey, Alasdair Breckenridge, Patrick Bye, Max Elstein, Ken Fotherby, and Tom Meade among others. I thank the

International Planned Parenthood Federation (IPPF) and Philip Kestelman in particular for help with the World directory of pill names. The IPPF Wall Chart 'The regulation of fertility' is acknowledged as source material for Figure 19. Figure 2 is reprinted from *International Family Planning Perspectives*, Vol. 5, No. 1 (1979), with permission of the Alan Guttmacher Institute.

My publishers have been most understanding, and I am particularly grateful to Adam Sisman, Hilary Dickinson, Nicola Bion, Angus Phillips, Hilary Feldman, and Peter Clifford for their editorial assistance.

The wisdom in this book comes from many sources. Not all can be mentioned, but all are thanked; and the author must be held responsible for any errors which remain.

Reviewers of the first edition made somewhat contradictory comments: some said that the book would be frightening, some that it displayed a 'pro-pill' bias. Perhaps this suggests that the balance was roughly right. I have been guided throughout by two principles: accuracy about what is known, and honesty about what is still unknown. I deny any conscious bias that would lead to the rejection or watering down of unpalatable facts, of which there are plenty in this book. In making decisions about oral contraception, all the relevant facts must be considered: the benefits as well as the risks of the pill, the risks avoided by taking it (chiefly those of pregnancy) and the risks of the available alternatives. If you read Chapter 6 'The pill in perspective' with an open mind in context with the other chapters, I think you will find that the facts speak for themselves: the pill *is* an appropriate choice for many women – but certainly not for all. A complete consideration of the facts can hardly fail to make anyone pro the pill, at least at their request for those I have called 'the safer women' – primarily healthy young women who do not smoke cigarettes. But there are other methods available even for them.

Never forget that you have a choice.

Some readers will disagree with my opinions or policies, and this is fine. There is still so much we do not yet know, experts disagree about how much weight to give to the facts that are known, and new facts may well emerge after publication. So much depends on people's attitudes, life-styles, and religious beliefs. Indeed, these issues warrant books of their own, and discussion of them and of other important topics has had to be brief.

Though one day there may be a usable male pill (see Chapter 9), I cannot, of course, write as a consumer . . . just as an understanding prescriber. Indeed, although the book is intended primarily for women considering or already taking the pill, I have been pleased to learn how many men have found it helpful.

Finally, I thank my parents for much guidance and practical help. And to my wife Gwyneth I owe an incalculable debt. Her advice and constructive criticism have been derived from practical experience, both as a family planning nurse and as a woman, a wife, and the mother of our three energetic children.

John Guillebaud, MA, FRCSE, FRCOG
Medical Director
Margaret Pyke Centre for Study and
Training in Family Planning

May 1984

Opinions on oral contraception vary – from those expressed by the Pill Victims' Action Group to those of many thousands of women who find it an excellent method of birth control. This book is based on evidence available at the time of writing.

Contents

How to use this book

The Pill can be read straight through, or dipped into as a reference book. You may well prefer to skip those sections marked with an asterisk (*) which are mainly for those who are interested in the finer details. But however you read it, be sure to include Chapter 6 which may help you to see 'the pill in perspective'.

Another possibility is to look first at the section '100 questions everyone asks about the pill' (page 229). The brief answer there may be all you need: but if you want a more detailed account the pages to read are also given.

Unless otherwise stated the word 'pill' on its own means the ordinary combined pill containing two hormones, an oestrogen and a progestogen, as explained in Chapter 2.

You, your doctor and the pill

Doctors who still have a kind of 'God complex' and expect all their decisions to be taken on trust, with no discussion, will not like this book. I hope that there will be few such or at least that they refrain from telling people what method of family planning they should use. If the pill is the method in question, in most countries doctors and nurses do the advising and the supplying, but they should not do the *deciding*: *that is your right.*

Nonetheless, even the most human and communicative doctors are unlikely to appreciate being told that you read in this or any other book what they should do next in your case! Make allowances for the fact that your clinic or family doctor has much experience, and may have very good reasons for disagreeing with something suggested here. The golden rule is, if you are ever in doubt about any aspect of pill-use, make sure that you talk things over with someone who knows the answers.

One problem shared by all doctors is lack of time. So I think most will be delighted if you are so well informed about the pill, having read this book, that by the time you come to their surgery or clinic you only have one or two points left to clear up.

And if the pill is not for you . . .

If the pill does not suit you, or if for some reason you must avoid or give up the pill, remember the choice is not between the pill and nothing; the coil (intra-uterine device: IUD), the cap (or diaphragm), and sheath can all provide very effective reversible contraception. There is another important possibility: the mini-pill, which in this book is referred to as the progestogen-only pill (POP) – see Chapter 8 for more details. And Chapter 10 gives a brief account of the other methods, including sterilization.

It is important to choose carefully, as the wrong choice can lead to problems; not least an unwanted pregnancy, either by using an inefficient method, or by using a better method inefficiently. The main reason why contraception seems such an unavoidable bore, or rather why it is so often avoided, is that all our present reversible methods are tried and found wanting in some way. They either have side-effects, or are a nuisance and interfere with love-making. So Chapter 9 deals with attempts to produce better methods for the future.

Introduction

by Gwyneth Guillebaud, SRN. ONC. FPA Cert.

Every day well over 50 million women reach out for a pill packet and swallow a tiny tablet which alters the course of their lives. About 150 million have done so at some time. And millions more will do so.

What that means to you – whether you are taking the pill yourself, have at some time taken it, or are thinking of doing so, whether you love someone who is taking it, or are in some other way involved or interested in oral contraceptives – what it means to all of us in fact is what this book is about.

The pill, very largely developed by men, produced by men, marketed by men, prescribed by men (written about by men!), and also undoubtedly of benefit to men, is taken by women. Should we as women be thankful? Twenty years ago when the pill became available, first in America, then elsewhere, that question would have been very much easier to answer. It seemed that at last there was an answer to the prayer of so many couples through the ages – contraception without complication. Simple and safe. The publicity was enormous, expectations were high.

What now, after two decades? *Should* we be thankful? Many of us, feminists and non-feminists alike, who have come to see control of fertility as a necessity, a right, and a freedom, would now like to respond by asking further questions. Is the price for this freedom too high? Does taking the pill mean taking control or being controlled? Moreover, who has gained the freedom? Has the pill liberated men more than women? It is hard to deny that many men have come to *assume* that women will take it. Why won't they take their own share of responsibility?

The pill has not lived up to all expectations, and women have become understandably cautious. There have been numerous press articles on the risks of the pill, and although many were unjustifiably scary, others were accurate. They have given some cause to question the medical safety of the pill method.

But if that is the case, why do so many women continue to reach regularly for the pill packet? There are several good

3

reasons. Being an ostrich is not one of them. What is needed is a balance of healthy caution and practical common sense. The best reason for taking the pill is that it works. Whatever else experience has shown, it has proved that oral contraception is easy and effective. Secondly, once stripped of sensationalism, the weight of informed opinion is that the risks relate to a very small number of women. Over the years it has become much easier to single out those who are at particular risk, and the doses used in current pills are much reduced and believed to be correspondingly safer.

Whatever the range of opinions about the pill, many women in modern society consider it a necessity. At an everyday and practical level, it has relieved millions of women from the constant fear of unwanted pregnancy. For all those who do experience side-effects, there are many who take it without problems and with great relief that a major aspect of their lives is no longer a source of stress. Our grandmothers were less fortunate.

Yet the introduction to the first edition of *The Pill* mentioned a British survey which revealed that of 1,000 women using the pill, one in three felt her health was being damaged and not properly monitored.

I can readily sympathize with those women – writing as a woman, with a woman's concerns about my body and the impact on it of contraception, and particularly the pill. As a contraceptive user, I have tried all the recommended reversible methods with a record of success and occasional failure, of overall satisfaction, but also of having to live with some side-effects.

To reject all contraception or use very unsafe methods, as some couples do, simply because the ideal method does not exist, is to put the clock right back. That is not freedom. We should avoid having unrealistic expectations. Almost nothing in life is completely safe and free of all health risks. Like every drug that has ever been devised, the pill can cause side-effects. However, when I took it I reminded myself that the betting odds were overwhelmingly in my favour.

Although every one of our current methods of family planning has one snag or another, I have proved like many other women that it is possible to find an acceptable method for every stage of our life. Of course I am lucky, having a husband who is

4

particularly well informed! But, just as important as the information, is a good relationship, the freedom to discuss one's feelings and fears. The eventual decision should ideally be a joint one.

Nevertheless if the method is one to be used by a woman, then the woman should make the final decision. The weight of medical opinion believes that for many women the known advantages of the pill far outweigh any possible risks. But it is for the individual woman to decide whether she can be confident it is really right for her – whatever a doctor, or family planning nurse, or anyone else may say. She must weigh up many considerations: how big a risk of pregnancy might be accepted, how easy the method is, the likelihood and nature of side-effects, the acceptability of other alternatives, and personal preferences. We live our lives and base our decisions on what we know, and the best and right decisions are those for which we feel we have taken responsibility.

That is why accurate knowledge is essential. The introduction to the first edition described this book as 'a handbook for the owner/driver of a healthy pill-taking body'. That is still the approach.

The facts as far as they are known are here. They may confirm your doubts about the pill. They may equally give you new confidence in it. It is up to you now to make the decisions.

G. M. G.

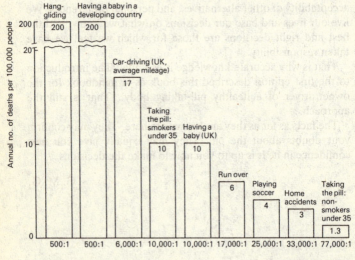

Fig. 1 Number of deaths per year for 100,000 people at risk
Notes: The implications of this figure are discussed on pages 143–4. The risk for pill-taking in non-smokers under 35 concerns circulatory diseases: for cancer, as explained on pages 120–3 the benefits tend to cancel the adverse effects, and the net resultant risk cannot yet be estimated.

1

Sex and contraception yesterday, today, and everywhere

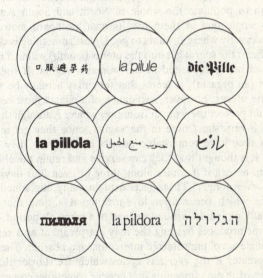

口服避孕药 la pilule die Pille

la pillola حبوب منع الحمل ピル

ПИЛЮЛЯ la píldora הגלולה

Fig. 2

The pill has spread far and wide throughout the world. It is no exaggeration to say that it has changed the course of recent history: not so much directly as indirectly by subtle changes in people's thinking, attitudes, and behaviour.

This first chapter covers a few subjects which are connected with or affected by the pill. They all deserve a mention, indeed each could have had a whole book devoted to it. If your appetite is whetted see Further reading (page 257).

Human fertility and the history of contraception

We break no records in the animal kingdom, but we are a remarkably fertile species. Doctors and others who work in family planning rapidly develop a great respect for human sperm! First seen under the microscope 300 years ago, they were initially thought to be 'parasites'. It was not until the 1840s that it was realized that they were crucial to the whole process of fertilization and the creation of a new individual. Millions of them are released at every act of intercourse when the man reaches climax. If each sperm in a normal man's ejaculate were able to find an egg the resulting number of pregnancies would be enough to populate the whole of North and South America! Every single one of them has its own 'outboard motor' and knows exactly where it wants to go. Unless something is done to stop them, the sperm get into the uterus (womb) within a minute or so of being deposited in the woman's vagina. If she has a climax (an orgasm), it seems that they may actually be sucked into the uterus; however, avoidance of a climax most certainly does *not* protect the woman from pregnancy. Although they will die in a very short time in the vagina, once they get into the uterus they have remarkable powers of survival. They like it there: it is thought that they can survive and retain the ability to fertilize an egg if it comes along three or even four days later, rarely even longer. These facts explain many unplanned pregnancies which occur after love-making at a time that many people think is safe, around the end of a woman's period. When she later produces her egg she may get pregnant as a result of that single act of unprotected intercourse *days* earlier. The risk is even greater if she *ever* has cycles which are shorter than the average of 28 days, meaning that her egg sometimes comes early. Hence for many women it is wrong to claim that this so-called post-menstrual phase is part of the 'safe period' at all. It is not the time to make love without precautions, unless you want a baby.

As far as nature is concerned, intercourse is designed to produce babies and ensure the survival of the species. Sex is also exciting and pleasurable, and especially so between two people who really love and care for each other. This helps to ensure that pregnancies do happen, and that the babies will survive because food and shelter are provided by their parents (see page 22). But if nature had its way each fertile woman could have a baby every year or two from the age of about 15 to over 40. For a long time past this has seemed a bit too much of a good thing.

It is not surprising therefore that methods of preventing pregnancy have been looked for and often practised. Right from the start in many societies they appear to have been frowned on. One of the main reasons was the fact that a high birth rate was essential for survival of the species. Both infant and adult mortality were extremely high and large numbers of children had to be born simply to ensure that each generation replaced itself. Medical advances have now controlled many of the killing diseases of the past, so that in the twentieth century we are faced with the quite different problem of a population explosion. But at various times in the last three or four thousand years it has been said that family planning even within marriage is danger-ous, sinful, antisocial, a threat to posterity, a form of witch-craft . . . Doctors have been as confused as anyone. Speaking to the British Medical Association in 1878, a Dr Routh said that 'sexual fraudulency' (his name for contraception) using the sheath or female barriers or spermicides might cause in one or other sex a whole range of diseases. These included cancer, mania leading to suicide, general nervous prostration, mental decay, loss of memory, and intense cardiac palpitations.

Nevertheless, the search for birth control methods continued. The earliest workers were highly unscientific and the methods they came up with were frequently useless, often uncomfortable, and sometimes ridiculous. In 1850 BC the Petri Papyrus from Egypt described the use of crocodile dung made into a paste and put into the vagina, or alternatively, a mixture whose chief ingredient was honey. Other nasty brews which could in fact have been effective as barriers and sometimes also because of their sperm-killing effects, included cabbage, pitch, ox gall, and elephant dung, to be used 'alone or in combination'. This was favoured by one Rhazes who died in about AD 923. A later Arab report suggested the use of the right testicle of a wolf wrapped in oil-soaked wool! There is not much point in trying to list all the confused ideas. But it is interesting that some of the myths which some people still believe today have a very long history. Soranos, who wrote during the second century AD, suggested

9

that the woman should 'hold back' (i.e. avoid having an orgasm) to prevent semen entering her uterus. She should then get up, sneeze, and drink something cold. Rhazes said something similar and added that she should jump backwards seven or nine times in order to dislodge the semen.

However, again from the earliest times, the ideal method was felt to be an *oral* contraceptive, which would avoid the need for doing something artificial and messy at the time of intercourse itself. In ancient China women were advised to swallow twenty-four live tadpoles in the early spring and they would then have five years free of conception. Albert the Great in the Middle Ages suggested bees should be eaten rather than tadpoles, an oral method with some pretty obvious side-effects . . . North African tribes once drank a gunpowder solution made with the foam gathered from the sweating flanks of their camels. None of these methods is likely actually to have worked, and some such as those based on arsenic or strychnine probably saw off more women than sperm! However, there were various potions based on plants; the Greek herbals of the first few centuries AD mentioned many. Anthropologists have accumulated from the folklore of primitive peoples all over the world the names of literally hundreds of plants which are believed to prevent or interrupt pregnancy. They have been made up into a variety of concoctions, often referred to as bush teas, and it is possible that a very few may really have had the desired effect. Some of the plants have been shown to contain oestrogens and so could have worked in the same sort of way as the pill (see Chapter 2). Others may have worked through alkaloids and similar substances not yet identified, either to stop fertilization or to cause abortion by contractions of the uterus. Indeed, research workers believe that somewhere in the world, in among the mumbo-jumbo, there may be a plant medicine in use from time immemorial which could provide the clue to a new and safe oral contraceptive. The World Health Organization has a Task Force looking into plant products for this very reason.

There is one plant which is very relevant to family planning right now, and that is the *Dioscorea* plant. This is a wild yam vine which clings to trees in the mountains of southern Mexico. Its coal-black roots are harvested by the Mexican Indians and used to produce the substance diosgenin, which was formerly the source of most of the hormones required for making pills. Recently there has been a world shortage of these yams, aggravated by the fact that they have never been successfully cultivated. So increasingly, alternative methods for making the hormones are now being used. (The modern history of the development of oral contraception for women is described in the next chapter).

Going back to the Ancients, oral contraception for the male was not entirely neglected. For instance, a man called Aetios, who wrote in the sixth century AD, recommended the burned testicles of the mule, drunk with a decoction of willow. The mule may well have been chosen because it is of course a sterile animal. In Chapter 9 I shall be considering research to produce rather more effective oral contraceptives for men.

The pill and the world scene

In recent years the birth rate in Western industrialized countries has fallen dramatically. The situation in much of the rest of the world is very different. It used to be said: 'There is one born every second.' In fact this is now very out of date. In round terms, based on the latest figures of the Population Reference Bureau, Washington DC, every 10 seconds 44 people are born on to this planet of ours. In the same time, 17 adults or children die. The difference means that 27 extra individuals have to be accommodated every 10 seconds (i.e. 2.7 per second), or the occupants of 500 full jumbo jets every day. World population is doubling every 39 years.

It has taken perhaps 10,000 years since agriculture was first practised for the population of the world to reach its present total of 4,800 million. If the same number again are to arrive in the next 39 years, and we are going to meet their most basic needs even as *badly* as we do for our present world, then we are going to have to double *everything*. For every house in the world we will need another house; for every school another school; for every hospital another hospital. Another world's worth of people will require at least as much again of food and clothing as is available now to the world of the early 1980s. A pretty daunting prospect: especially when you add three further facts.

First, there is no humane way that at least one further doubling can be avoided. The parents of all these new people are

11

already born. Of the world's population 34 per cent is under the age of 15 and in most developing countries the figure is 40–50 per cent. If by some miracle Mr and Mrs World Citizen had on average only the number of children required for replacement (a little over two), starting tomorrow, the population of the whole world would still not stabilize until there were more than 9,000 million people.

Second, birth rates, although falling in most countries in the developing world, are in fact a very long way above the replacement level. For this reason we may have to contemplate four or even eight times the present population of the world. Unless, that is, nature's most unwelcome solution to the imbalance between birth rates and death rates occurs on a large enough scale: i.e. a massive increase in the number of deaths, which could be due to famine, epidemics, or of course wars.

Third, and most important, two-thirds of the people in the world even now lack a bare minimum of the requirements for reasonable health and comfort. Fifteen million children die each year before the age of 5, partly from malnutrition. Suppose the impossible were achieved in the next 39 years and all the requirements of the world were doubled as just described. Unless the present unjust and unequal distribution of the world's wealth – itself a great wrong – were also put right at each level of need, the *percentage* of deprived people would remain unchanged. With a doubling of world numbers that would mean *twice as many* destitute as there are now.

Nothing I have just said is particularly new and the facts must be known to the politicians and rulers of most countries of the world. Yet there is far too much windy rhetoric and not enough appropriate action. These matters are very complex with absolutely no easy solutions.

We human beings have difficulty in appreciating things on a large scale. 'The death of one baby is a tragedy – the death of millions is a statistic.' We too rarely consider what happens when the things we do as individuals are also done by millions of other individuals. For example, 'My car is my car – everybody else's car is "traffic".' 'My visit to the seaside is my holiday – everybody else is a "tripper".' And, 'My baby is my baby – everybody else's baby is "over-population".'

It is not by any means just a numbers game. There are other

12

serious, interrelated problems facing the world which are discussed in many books (*e.g. Only One Earth* – see Further reading). These include depletion of resources – oil is the obvious example, but the pressure on many others such as the habitats for wild creatures, fisheries, forests, grass- and crop-lands increases all the time, due in part to excessive consumption; damage to the environment through pollution of many kinds (nuclear wastes being perhaps the most worrying of all); not to mention terrorism, forced migration of whole populations, the armaments race, and so on.

Roughly speaking, every new birth in 'over-developed' countries like Britain and America will lead during the lifetime of that person to something between twenty and forty times more impact on the environment than a new arrival in a poor country like, say, Bangladesh. This is because each of us in the rich countries is like a cog in a machine which eats up raw materials of all kinds at one end, and spews out rubbish at the other. On this basis, 'over-population' is by no means just a problem for the poor countries as we may like to think.

Yet it is too simple to suggest that the solution is to stabilize or reduce the population of the rich as well as the poor countries of the world. Many other changes are necessary including, a lot of people would believe, substantially more effective help for the less developed countries by the rich ones; and rejection of the often wasteful and dehumanizing philosophy that 'Biggest is best'. Much better slogans are: 'Small is beautiful' and 'Enough is enough' – see books with these titles (page 260).

'The rich get richer and the poor get children'

Partly because methods like the pill are readily available and so much more efficient than the older family planning methods, birth rates in the over-developed countries are uniformly low, mostly around or below replacement level. This is to be welcomed.

Why, with a few exceptions, are most of the less developed countries still so far from stabilizing their population numbers? An important reason is that the pill and other effective methods of family planning are in practice *not* available to so many who need them. The World Fertility Survey found almost 50 per cent

13

of married women in the developing world wanted no more children. But they nearly all lacked access to the methods that would enable them to avoid having more. They need better methods, more effectively distributed, so that every couple in the world can use them if they so wish – as a human right, let alone for population reasons. Because there are so few doctors, especially in country areas, a committee of international experts has said, 'Whoever normally meets the health needs of the community, whether doctor, nurse, traditional midwife, pharmacist or store-keeper would be an appropriate person to distribute oral contraceptives, supported by adequate information, education and medical back-up services.' This idea of using non-doctors to distribute the pill is very controversial: it should be discussed in the light of the relative risks of unplanned pregnancy in the community concerned (see 'The Pill off Prescription', Further reading).

Motivation to use the methods is equally important. One reason why methods of family planning are not always effectively used in many poor countries, even when they are available, is that the death rate among children is so high. Parents tend to play safe and so have more children on average than would be required strictly to replace themselves. They also *need* more children. As an ancient proverb puts it, a child has 'one mouth, but two hands'. The work done in the household by either a son or a daughter is more obviously valuable than the extra food he or she eats. And in the absence of any social security schemes, children are literally vital as 'insurance' for one's old age.

These are very complex problems. There are formidable obstacles to be overcome: superstitions, rigid social and religious traditions, and outdated male-dominant attitudes among them. Under-privileged and minority groups can become suspicious of what they describe as racialism, elitism, or genocide disguised as family planning. Any solution must provide the various methods of birth control, improve the status of women, and be combined with social and economic development of the right kind which benefits all, rather than just a rich minority. This means making available so-called 'appropriate' technology (the pill itself comes under this heading) in the villages and slums of the less developed countries, along with improved nutrition, health care – especially for mothers and babies – housing, and education.

Organizations such as Oxfam and Tear Fund have shown for some time now how things should be done. Population Concern, the Conservation Society, and Friends of the Earth are other organizations worthy of support. They are concerned to preserve a habitable environment for all the world's children, as well as for other species sharing the planet (see Useful addresses, page 265, for Britain).

A final thought: it has been said, and it is probably true, that more babies are prevented worldwide by breast-feeding than by all the world's family planning programmes put together. What this statement means is that if almost all women in a community do breast-feed their children, their overall fertility is reduced. Certainly, if breast-feeding becomes infrequent – a most unwelcome trend in many areas – the interval between children is much shorter. This does not contradict the well-known fact that if individual couples rely solely on breast-feeding for family planning, they are liable to be let down. This is because to have a really good contraceptive effect, breast-feeding must be inten-sive, as practised traditionally in many developing countries: the baby must receive no supplementary feeds.

But the second point which emerges from the statement is that present family planning programmes are most inadequate. Worldwide, each year there are about 40 million induced abortions, of which half are illegal. These are believed to lead to the death of something between 20,000 and 200,000 women each year; and many more are made permanently infertile. This is proof that, even in their present circumstances, people do want fewer children. Far too many, for many different kinds of reasons, would welcome, and are not being given, the tools for the job: including the pill.

The pill and women's role in society

'The pill has fallen from its pedestal to take its place among the other contraceptives, each with flaws and assets . . . [But] without the advent of the pill and women's response to the freedom it *promised*, our present age would clearly be very different, and so would our vision of the future.' (Susan Scrimshaw, *Family Planning Perspectives*, 1982.)

In some countries, mostly but not exclusively less developed, the status of women has to be improved before much headway can be made in introducing the idea of family limitation by any methods. But it is also true that in many other societies the pill, above all other methods of family planning, has helped to bring about big changes in the role of women. This is because, for the first time, women have the option to decide how many children to have, when to have them, and whether to have them at all. Now they no longer necessarily have to be constantly child-bearing and child-rearing. Marriage and the first child can be and are delayed (this can be overdone, however, see page 109). Women are free to proceed to higher education and to pursue independent careers far more than in the past. There is still a long way to go, however, and many job and other opportunities are still not available to women. So it is probably no coincidence that the pill has been widely available for the last fifteen years in most Western countries, and over the same period movements for women's rights and equal opportunities have become more effective.

Some women of course still prefer their main role in life to be that of wife and mother. They should not feel inferior for not aspiring to be engineers or Prime Ministers. Neither should the aspiring engineers feel bad for not opting for parenthood. The right to choose is the main thing and this exists far more now than in the days before the pill.

Nature was very unkind in placing so very many of the problems connected with having babies on the one sex. Problems with the sexual apparatus of women can happen at any time, particularly at puberty and through the fertile years (pre-menstrual tension, painful or heavy periods, and all the troubles of child-bearing), at the menopause, and even in old age. Men, on the other hand, get off virtually scot-free, with nothing to worry about apart from a bit of prostate trouble and that usually not until they are past the age of 70. The pill has helped to even out this imbalance between the sexes: not only by its obvious effect in reducing the frequency and hence the risks of child-bearing, but also because it so commonly improves the symptoms of the menstrual cycle. But the pill for women also has many drawbacks, of course. So even more welcome will be the day when a male pill is available, so that men can take

16

more of a share in the whole business of family planning (see Chapter 9).

Usage of the pill in the world – and in the United Kingdom

The proportion of pill-users in each country of the world varies enormously and most of the estimates are very unreliable. Usage in most of the less developed countries is relatively low for the reasons given earlier. But even in countries without those obstacles, the proportion of women using the pill can be low, depending on the alternatives available, and sometimes for religious reasons (as in Italy or Ireland) or for reasons of medico-politics. According to one estimate in 1977, under 2 per cent of women aged 15 to 44 were pill-users in Greece and less than 1 per cent in Japan. Yet in the Netherlands the rate that year was over 40 per cent.

The United Kingdom is an example of a country where the pill is still, in spite of many worrying newspaper articles, the commonest method being used at any one time, as shown in Figure 3. The proportion of women under 30 using it is of course much higher than the average 26 per cent figure. In recent surveys around 70 per cent of sexually active women in their twenties said that they were on the pill. On the other hand, over the age of 30 sterilization is becoming so popular that, if current trends continue, in the majority of couples one or other of the partners will have been sterilized by the time the wife is 35.

In Figure 3, it is a bit disturbing that 15 per cent – one seventh of the total – do not appear to be using a recognized method of birth control and yet are not trying to become pregnant. Some may be abstaining from intercourse but many are not. In a recent report, more than a quarter of couples who married between 1971 and 1975 admitted risking pregnancy before their marriage by using no method at all or 'sometimes taking a chance'. A similar amount of risk-taking doubtless continues today, and in other countries as well as in the United Kingdom.

Unwanted pregnancy

'Most accidents are caused by a human and most humans are caused by an accident.' Thanks to the pill this is less true than it

17

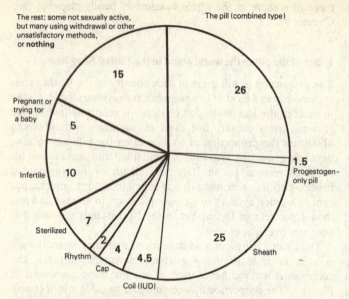

The rest: some not sexually active, but many using withdrawal or other unsatisfactory methods, or **nothing**

The pill (combined type)

15

26

Pregnant or trying for a baby

5

1.5
Progestogen-only pill

Infertile

10

7

Sterilized

2

Rhythm

4

Cap

4.5

Coil (IUD)

25

Sheath

Fig. 3 How the methods are used in the United Kingdom of Great Britain and Northern Ireland (based on FPA estimates, December 1982)

Note: The percentages shown are out of a total of about 11.5 million women in the 'fertile age-group' (15–44).

once was. Every year, however, there are still quite a number of first births that occur within eight months of marriage, and it is known that a high percentage of parents, particularly with large families, did not plan their latest arrival. The number of requests for termination of pregnancy (abortion) is another sign of the same problem. Being pregnant when you do not want to be is a good recipe for guilt feelings and much personal misery, not to mention family rows and money crises. It is not impossible, of course, for an unwanted pregnancy to lead eventually to the birth of a wanted, loved, and well-cared-for child. However, this may well not be the outcome.

I am sure there is no need to dwell on this point. You would not be reading this book if you were not already convinced that children should come by loving choice rather than careless chance.

The pill and sexually transmitted diseases

I considered the 'population explosion' earlier but there is another recent phenomenon, the 'copulation explosion'. If the effects of the former seem a bit remote, those of the latter can be a bit too close for comfort. An increasing number of people nowadays expect more sex more often and with less commitment. Three pretty obvious statements can be made about this. First, couples where 'a one-man woman sleeps only with her one-woman man' never catch any truly sexually transmitted disease (STD, or venereal disease, as it used to be called). Second, the pill does make it easier to have sex in a casual way, perhaps with less commitment. Third, the pill has tended to replace the sheath, and the sheath is quite an effective barrier to the catching or passing on of STDs.

The pill offers some protection against some types of STD, but not enough (page 103); it is thus often blamed for the epidemic the world is now experiencing. To the extent that it has removed one of the important deterrents to copulation without commitment to your partner – fear of unwanted pregnancy – there must be some truth in this. But how keen we always are to find a scapegoat for the ills of society. The pill does not *cause* STDs, people do, by catching them from each other.

It is a very common myth that people who get these diseases were not careful enough in choosing their partner; and that if you are particularly 'clean' and 'choosy' you will be able to avoid them. Unfortunately, this is not so. STDs cross all geographical and social barriers. They can and do afflict Government Ministers, doctors, and nurses, just as much as dustmen, cleaners, and dockyard workers and their partners. You may in fact have been very selective as to your partner; but if he or she has had intercourse just once with someone infected with STD, then you too could be infected. Putting it another way, STDs are spread now not so much by the 'professional' as by the enthusiastic amateur.

Why do we no longer refer to 'venereal disease'?

This name is a bit old fashioned as it only refers officially to the two best-known diseases, syphilis and gonorrhoea, with (usually) the addition of one or perhaps two others, depending on the laws of the particular country. Yet the list of infections which can be transmitted in this way is increasing all the time and at the last count there were about 25. They are now nearly as common as respiratory infections (such as colds and influenza). Some of them are almost never caught any other way than by sexual contact. Others, such as a particular form of liver disease (hepatitis), can be caught through sex, though the infection is often passed on in other ways.

What are the symptoms of sexually transmitted diseases?

One of the main problems is that the diseases frequently cause no symptoms at all, especially in women. This means that no one should wait for symptoms before seeking advice if they know, or discover, that they have been exposed to this risk. A *vaginal discharge* in the woman, or a discharge from the *penis* in the man, are the two commonest symptoms. If a woman discovers that her male partner has a discharge, then she has very likely also picked up a form of STD and both partners should go to a clinic. A vaginal discharge in a woman, on the other hand, could have a different explanation.

In women, *pain in the lower abdomen*, severe but different from period pains and specially bad with love-making, can be due to pelvic infection (which is often due to STD) whether or not there is also a discharge. *If in doubt, if either has taken a risk, both partners should seek advice*, ideally from a clinic which specializes in these diseases, if there is one in your locality (see Useful addresses, page 261). Treatment is entirely confidential, and you do not require a letter of referral from your doctor.

Urethritis can also occur in both sexes. This means inflammation of the tube which conveys urine from the bladder, and is one cause of a *burning pain* on passing water. This does not necessarily mean a sexual infection; it is more likely if the symptom occurs in a man, or in either sex if there is also a discharge.

The fourth most common symptom is a *sore or ulcer*, on the penis in the male, or in the vagina or outside on the vulva in the female. Such sores can be painful if due to the herpes virus, a modern scourge causing recurrent attacks which are infectious each time. A painless sore must on no account be disregarded as it could be due to the most serious STD, syphilis. *Warts* on the genitals can also be acquired sexually.

20

Discharges, sores, and warts can sometimes cause some irritation or itching but the symptoms may be so minimal that there is a great temptation to do nothing about them. For the sake of your future health and, in women, because pelvic infections due to gonorrhoea and other STDs can sometimes block up your uterine tubes and so prevent you ever having a baby, it is essential not to attempt any form of self-treatment. Take expert advice if there is the slightest doubt. You may only notice vaginal warts. But at the same time as catching these, you could, without realizing it, have acquired something more serious like gonorrhoea. Six out of ten women with such warts were found to have some other STD as well; and half of all women with gonorrhoea have no symptoms. It is also essential to continue to the end of any course of treatment, even if you feel well; to report any new symptoms such as *rashes*; to have all the tests recommended: and to help the clinic to trace any contacts.

Last but not least, remember that there is no immunity after an attack of most STDs. You can be cured of gonorrhoea in the morning with the right antibiotic treatment and catch it again the same evening. But the good news is that with early and correct treatment almost all sexually transmitted infections are entirely curable. See Further reading for more details (page 257).

It is very interesting that research is now suggesting that cancer of the cervix (entrance to the uterus) behaves rather like an STD. The main microscopic type of this cancer never occurs in a woman who has not had intercourse. It is far more common in women who have sex first when they are very young (under the age of 16) and who have had many different partners. *If this applies to you, or if you have had herpes or wart virus infections* (also risk factors), *do not panic*. Nature gives an early warning of future trouble, which can be found in cervical smears (page 67). Actual cancer is then preventable by minor treatment, usually as an out-patient. Even if in your area the policy is for routine smears at least every five years (one system being around age 20, 25, 30, 35, etc.), you should ask the doctor in confidence whether to have them more often because of your sexual history.

The pill and responsibility in sex

Some people think that the only things that show whether

somebody has been sexually responsible are if he or she has (a) not caused an unwanted pregnancy and (b) not acquired a sexually transmitted disease. Both are worthwhile aims – a little negative perhaps, but good. Yet the good can sometimes be an enemy of the best. Making love is something special, definitely not for throwing around. It is nature's physical 'seal of approval' on a loving and caring relationship between two people. Deep down, everyone knows that a sexual experience which pre-dates a loving experience is a pale shadow of the real thing. Many can confirm that love-making is actually more fun and more exciting if the couple care for and trust each other: if in fact they are 'in love'. Love says 'What can I give?' much more than 'What can I get?' *As a minimum*, I think that responsible sex means asking these three questions before any couple make love: 'Do we want, and can we care for, a baby?', 'If not, are we using a reliable method of family planning, such as the pill?'; and most important, 'Will making love with this person lead to anyone, my partner, myself, or any third party, being hurt?' Having realized that someone might very well get hurt, some couples actually decide not to have sex even with precautions. They are using, if you like, what has been described as the 'safest of all oral contraceptives', namely the word 'No' . . . Worth a thought: though clearly abstinence will not seem a relevant suggestion to most people today.

The pill cannot be expected to be a cure-all of society's ills. Nor should it be blamed for too many of them – they are caused by people, not by the pill. It can certainly enable some people to behave irresponsibly, people who forget that bodies also have feelings and emotions attached. Even then, at least a disastrous pregnancy will be avoided. A child has the best chance in life if born to parents who trust each other and are prepared to keep *working* on their relationship, so as to ensure an emotionally secure and happy home for all the years he or she needs to reach maturity.

I believe that pill prescribers, whatever their own religious and moral views, should meet and counsel the person or couple requesting contraception on their own ground. Consider the following analogy. If I were a Jehovah's Witness, it would be immoral for me to receive a blood tranfusion. Yet, as a doctor, I could feel that it was right for me to transfuse a dangerously ill patient who did not share my views.

Thus prescribers of the pill need not betray their own principles while refraining from forcing them on others. They should have come to terms with their own sexuality and should be as good at listening as at talking, though prepared to say a 'word in season' based on the first paragraph of this section if (and only if) appropriate. They should be equipped to give helpful counselling, particularly for those who are immature, emotionally, whatever their age in years. Prescribers should be specially sensitive too to those with inhibitions of whatever kind, for example some who may have guilt feelings about sex, or about family planning. Everyone is different.

2

The pill: how does it work?

The idea of an oral contraceptive has been around for at least two thousand years. But nothing very useful came out of centuries of magic and mumbo-jumbo plus a great deal of trial and error. It was only when the normal processes of male and female reproduction were better understood that scientists could begin to devise more effective methods for blocking them.

The normal menstrual cycle

During their fertile years women are unique in having a more or less regular cycle of changes in their bodies. This cycle is caused by the ebb and flow in the bloodstream of various hormones or chemical messengers which are released into it by certain glands. The whole process is controlled by the brain, as is shown by the well-known fact that if a woman has a stressful emotional upset her periods can stop altogether for months at a time. Parts of the brain which are particularly involved have special names (such as the preoptic area and the hypothalamus), but I shall here call them simply the 'base of the brain'.

As you can see in Figure 4, just below the base of the brain is the pituitary gland, sometimes called the 'leader of the hormone orchestra' because it is so important. Yet it is really quite small, just the size of a large pea. The ovaries and uterus are the other main parts of the system and are also shown. Blood flows through them all connecting the whole system together. Any hormone released into the blood by one gland can therefore travel to all the others and can cause its own specific effects there or as appropriate anywhere in the whole body.

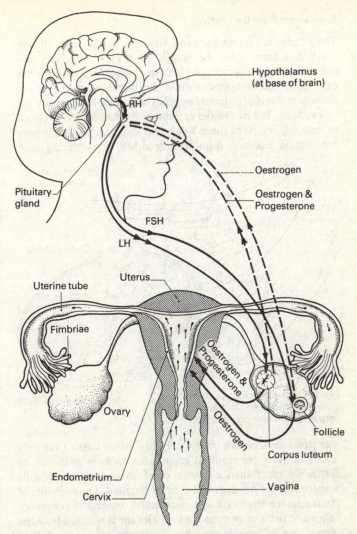

Fig. 4 The female reproductive system: control of the menstrual cycle

Notes: 1. Single arrowhead ▶ relates to events of the first half of the cycle (follicular phase). Double arrowheads ▶▶ relate to the second half (luteal phase).

2. Dotted lines show feedback effects (see page 31).

3. RH = releasing hormone   FSH = follicle stimulating hormone
   LH = luteinising hormone.

Egg-release from the ovaries

The ovaries are about the same size as a peach-stone, though much less hard. Like the testicle of a man they have two functions: the production and release of special sex cells (in this case eggs) and of hormones into the bloodstream. There are literally millions of potential egg cells in the ovaries of a baby girl before birth, but by the age of puberty the number has dropped to only 200,000. Yet there will be no shortage. Normally only one egg is released from one or other ovary during each

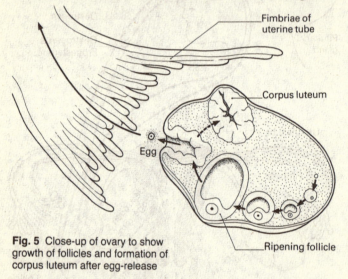

Fig. 5 Close-up of ovary to show growth of follicles and formation of corpus luteum after egg-release

menstrual cycle which commonly lasts for 28 days. Thus only about thirteen are required each year. As no woman can be fertile for more than a maximum of about forty years, only something over 500 eggs will ever be required. Occasionally, of course, more than one egg is released, leading if pregnancy follows to twins or perhaps triplets. The egg is released from the largest out of several fluid-filled balloons or egg-sacs called follicles and is picked up by the seaweed-like fronds (or fimbriae) of the outer end of one of the uterine (Fallopian) tubes: see Figure 5. It then starts its journey down the uterine tube, partly by the whole tube contracting and partly because there are microscopic paddles (cilia) within it which beat rhythmically in the direction of the uterus.

This happens about the middle of a cycle, if it is going to be 4 weeks in length. The time from egg-release (often called ovulation) to the start of the next period is the only part of the cycle which is fixed in length and lasts 14 days. Many quite normal cycles last less or more than the usual 28 days. If so the variability is almost all in the length of the first phase of the cycle from the start of the period up to egg-release. The first day of menstrual bleeding is always called day 1 of the cycle. So if, for example, a woman has a 35-day cycle, egg-release happens on day (35−14 =) 21.

The cycle occurs because of a marvellously controlled interaction of hormones. The most important ones are two produced by the pituitary gland – follicle stimulating hormone (FSH) and luteinising hormone (LH) – and two from the ovaries – oestrogen and progesterone. Up to the time of egg-release, the ovary produces only the one female hormone called oestrogen. It is made in cells within the walls of the follicles, depicted in Figure 5. These give their name to the first part of the cycle – the follicular phase. During the second part of the menstrual cycle, for almost exactly 14 days, the particular empty follicle from which the egg came that month now produces another hormone called progesterone as well as oestrogen. It also turns yellow in colour, and so is given the name corpus luteum (which just means 'yellow body' in Latin), and this part of the cycle is called the luteal phase (see Figure 6a). The name luteinising hormone for the hormone which causes this change means no more than 'the yellow-making hormone'.

The uterus

These hormones travel to the uterus during both phases of the cycle. Their main business there is to thicken its lining with extra glandular tissue and blood-vessels so that it is ready just in case a pregnancy starts that month. If the woman has recently had unprotected sex, a sperm may reach the egg in the uterine tube and join up with it. This is fertilization. The fertilized egg starts just 14 hundredths of a millimetre in size. It begins to divide on its journey along the uterine tube towards the uterus, and

27

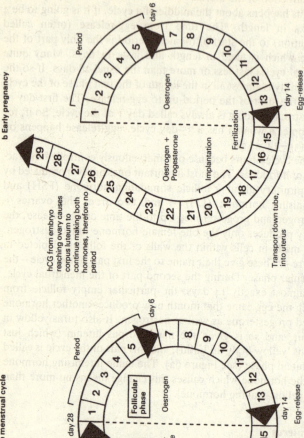

a The menstrual cycle

Period

day 6

Follicular phase

Oestrogen

day 14

Egg-release

Luteal phase

Oestrogen + Progesterone

day 28

Rapid fall in level of two hormones from the ovary causes period

b Early pregnancy

Period

day 6

Oestrogen

day 14

Egg-release

Fertilization

Oestrogen + Progesterone

Implantation

Transport down tube, into uterus

hCG from embryo reaching ovary causes corpus luteum to continue making both hormones, therefore no period

Fig. 6 (a) The menstrual cycle (b) Early pregnancy. *Note:* Assumes standard 28-day cycle. Follicular phase is the part that varies, if the actual cycle is longer or shorter than 28 days.

embeds itself in the prepared lining around the nineteenth day of the cycle. This is called implantation (Figure 6b).

The embryo, as the early pregnancy is called, now has just over a week to prevent the next period happening. This is vital, otherwise it will be washed out by the menstrual flow. It does this by itself producing a special hormone, whose name is human chorionic gonadotrophin (hCG). This sends an urgent message in the bloodstream to the yellow body, the corpus luteum, to make sure it keeps on producing its hormones (oestrogen and progesterone). These therefore keep coming in the blood to the uterus, and ensure that the lining of the uterus is not shed, so it can continue to provide nourishment for the developing embryo (Figure 6b). Considering this intricate series of events, it is remarkable that a fully formed human being ever results.

Menstruation: the period

In fact, implantation very often fails – probably in over one-third of cases. See page 207. Or the egg was never fertilized. Either way, the preparations for pregnancy come to nothing. The ovary stops producing oestrogen and progesterone as regularly at about 14 days after egg-release as if it had a timing mechanism programmed to switch it off. This rapid loss of the hormones which produce and maintain the lining of the uterus causes it to break down and leave the body through the cervix and vagina (Figure 4). This causes the bleeding of the first day of the next period, which is day 1 of the *next* menstrual cycle (see Figure 6a).

The pituitary gland

Just as hormones from the ovary control what happens in the uterus, so the hormones from the pituitary gland tell the ovary to produce the correct hormones for each phase of the cycle. One of them, luteinising hormone (LH), is released in large amounts at mid-cycle, and this signal is what actually triggers off the bursting of the largest follicle to release an egg. This signal is never given in pregnancy because enough of the hormones oestrogen and progesterone comes from the ovary to the pituitary gland to 'switch it off'. This prevents any further eggs being released and so explains why a woman who is already pregnant cannot go on getting pregnancies in the next nine months.

The pill

The combined oral contraceptive pill contains similar hormones to the oestrogen and progesterone produced by the ovary. Hence the pituitary gland is, as you might say, 'fooled' into thinking the woman is already pregnant. From its point of view, there is no need to send out hormones to stimulate the ovaries if there are already high levels of ovarian-type hormones. So the pituitary cuts drastically its output of the hormones FSH and LH. In particular there are no more of those mid-cycle 'surges' of a large amount of LH which are essential for egg-release. With so little of the hormones from the pituitary reaching them, the ovaries also go into a resting state, and produce minimal amounts of natural oestrogen and progesterone. Both the pituitary and the ovaries are like factories where the main production line has stopped, perhaps for a works' holiday, but small-scale production and essential maintenance are continuing. Such a factory can start full-scale production at short notice as soon as the work-force returns. Similarly, when a woman discontinues the pill, the hormone factories in the pituitary and ovaries rapidly return to normal working.

While a woman is taking the pill the normal menstrual cycle stops altogether. However, 'periods' of a sort are still produced, because the artificial hormones in the pill do have some effect on the lining of the uterus. When they are removed for one week out of every four this rather thinner lining comes away along with some bleeding. See page 38 for more details about this.

So much for a brief summary of the menstrual cycle and how the pill works. Continue reading here if you would like a more detailed account, but otherwise you may like to move on to page 34.

* More about the menstrual cycle

* *The follicular phase*

In order to start each new cycle, a special hormone called the releasing hórmone (RH) travels from the base of the brain and causes the pituitary gland to release follicle stimulating hormone (FSH). See Figure 4; you will find it helpful to keep referring to this and to Figure 6 throughout this section. FSH travels in the blood to the ovaries. Its main action, as its name implies, is to stimulate the growth of some of the many thousands of follicles which are contained in each ovary. Follicles are tiny, thick-walled, fluid-filled egg-sacs, each lined by a layer of cells which are capable of producing hormones, and also containing an immature egg cell (oocyte). FSH usually stimulates about twenty of these follicles to grow, and also causes the lining cells to start to manufacture oestrogen and release it into the blood. One particular follicle in one or other ovary is stimulated to grow and to 'ripen' more than all the others. Its egg cell is also maturing, ready to be released and, should it get the chance, to be fertilized.

Oestrogens are the fundamentally female hormones which influence the whole body, producing rounded contours, breast development, and many other features of femininity. They also stimulate the uterus to grow its new lining to replace the one that was shed at the previous menstrual period. The lining is made of many little glands, set in several layers of cells which also contain arteries and veins. Oestrogen makes the glands grow and the layers of intervening cells increase.

Meanwhile the rising levels of oestrogen in the blood have been having a most important effect back on the base of the brain and the pituitary gland. This is known as 'negative feedback' and it is important to understand this if you are to understand clearly how the pill works.

In general terms, negative feedback means that if the level of a hormone in the blood goes *up*, the level of the stimulating hormone which *caused* it to go up is made to go *down*.

In the menstrual cycle, this means for example:

up ↑ oestrogen in blood causes *down* ↓ FSH

The opposite is also true:

down ↓ oestrogen in blood causes *up* ↑ FSH

Engineers call this a servo-mechanism.

So at the stage of the menstrual cycle we have now reached, the rise in the level of oestrogen causes over several days a fall in the pituitary gland's output of its FSH.

By about the thirteenth day of a standard 28-day cycle the stimulated follicles have produced a rise of oestrogen in the blood to a peak level up to six times higher than it was on the first day. By negative feedback this has caused the level of the stimulating hormone FSH to drop. Now a most interesting and crucially different thing happens. Once the amount of oestrogen reaching the pituitary gland gets to a critical level, it releases into the bloodstream a sudden surge of luteinising hormone (LH). In other words, the *rise* in oestrogen is now causing a *rise* of a hormone from the pituitary. This is called 'positive feedback', to distinguish it from the negative type which operates all the rest of the time throughout the menstrual cycle.

This large amount of LH is conveyed by the blood to the active ovary. This is the one containing the largest follicle, now a balloon bulging the surface of the ovary and about 2 centimetres in diameter. The main job of this surge of LH is to cause the balloon to burst, resulting in ovulation and the release of a now mature and fertilizable egg. If all goes well, this is picked up by the fimbriae of the uterine tube and transported towards the uterus (see Figure 5). As this occurs some women notice in their lower abdomen, on one or other side, a variable amount of pain which is given the German name Mittelschmerz.

Once the egg has been released, the follicle collapses and becomes that bright yellow body, the corpus luteum. Along with the change in colour of the cells lining its wall there is a change in what they do. As well as continuing to produce oestrogen, for the first time these luteal cells start to manufacture and release into the blood a new hormone called progesterone.

* *The luteal phase*

Progesterone, like oestrogen, has effects all over the body and, for instance, is responsible for the slight rise in body temperature during the second half of the cycle which is the basis for the temperature method of family planning. But its main effect is on the lining of the uterus, to prepare it for a pregnancy. Indeed the word progesterone means 'pro-gestation: in favour of child-bearing'. It thickens the lining of the uterus still further and causes its glands to release a nutritious fluid. After implantation, which if a sperm successfully fertilizes an egg is about five days after its release, the embryo produces hCG. This hormone exactly copies the action of LH from the pituitary (page 29) and so prolongs the life of the corpus luteum. This ensures that it

32

continues to produce sufficient progesterone and oestrogen. As long as these hormones continue to be produced by the ovary, there will be no menstrual flow and the embryo can remain secure within the lining of the uterus. A second effect of these two hormones, working in concert, is to lower the amounts of LH and FSH released from the pituitary by the more usual negative feedback process. This is important, as it prevents any more surges of LH.

If, however, a sperm fails to reach the egg on its way down the tube, the egg dies at a maximum of 48 hours after ovulation. For reasons which are still not clear, the corpus luteum abruptly ceases to function twelve to fourteen days after it was first formed, unless hCG from a developing embryo dictates differently. There is therefore a rapid fall in the levels of both oestrogen and progesterone. This has two results: first, by negative feedback, the amount of RH coming from the base of the brain to the pituitary increases and therefore the amount of FSH released increases. When this extra FSH in the blood reaches the ovaries, another group of twenty or so follicles are stimulated to grow, one of them being destined to release its egg during the *next* normal menstrual cycle. Second, the sudden fall in the levels of both oestrogen and progesterone in the bloodstream reaching the uterus causes local changes in its now thick lining which lead to it being shed during a normal menstrual period. How heavy and how long the bleeding during the first few days of the next cycle is varies considerably. Substances called prostaglandins are involved in this process: one of their effects is to ensure that the uterus contracts to expel the blood, but this can also cause menstrual cramping pain (dysmenorrhoea) which can be severe in some women.

The description I have just given is still simplified. 'Oestrogen' is in fact a family of hormones, the most important member of which in the menstrual cycle is oestradiol. The 'surge' of LH is accompanied by a smaller surge of FSH. Releasing hormone (RH) normally reaches the pituitary in an intermittent, so-called pulsatile fashion, and this important mechanism is disturbed by progesterone (or any progestogen). Another hormone from the pituitary gland called prolactin is involved; and the whole cycle can be affected by quite different hormones such as those from the thyroid gland, as well as by the nervous system.

How the pill was developed

To recap: so long as there are reasonably high levels of the two hormones oestrogen and progesterone, the base of the brain and the pituitary gland are kept inactive (by negative feedback). This prevents:

(a) release of sufficient FSH to ripen any follicles in preparation for egg-release;

(b) any surges of LH, without which the actual process of release of an egg is impossible.

These results are regularly produced by the high levels of both the natural hormones during the second half of the normal menstrual cycle and throughout any pregnancy.

That the corpus luteum of pregnancy stops further egg-release was first shown in the early 1900s. In 1921 the Austrian Dr Haberlandt was the first scientist on record to suggest that extracts from the ovaries of pregnant animals might be used as oral contraceptives. It was in fact from extracts of either the corpus luteum or the follicles of rat ovaries that progesterone and several different oestrogens were isolated and eventually each chemical formula was determined.

By the late 1930s Dr Rock and Dr Kurzrok in America, among others, were beginning to use the hormones in both fertile and infertile women. As Dr Haberlandt had predicted, and some researchers using rabbits had shown, these hormones could be used to stop egg-release.

However, natural progesterone and oestrogens were not satisfactory when given by mouth since they are largely destroyed in the digestive system. In these experiments they had to be given by injection. In 1939 Inhoffen in Germany managed to produce an oestrogen which could be taken orally. It was called ethinyloestradiol, but over 20 years were to pass before it became one of the two oestrogens used in combined pills. The other is called mestranol.

The other main problem in the 1930s and early 1940s was that the raw material for all steroid hormones had to be extracted from animal sources. To produce just 12 milligrams of oestradiol, for example, required the ovaries of 80,000 sows. This made the hormones fearfully expensive. The next breakthrough came in 1943 when an eccentric American chemist called Russell Marker managed to produce pure progesterone from diosgenin extracted from wild Mexican yams.

Using the same raw material, a team led by George Rosenkranz and Carl Djerassi then produced the first orally active progestogen, norethisterone, in 1951. In North America this is known as norethindrone, and it remains perhaps the most widely used progestogen to this day. Working independently, two years later Dr Frank Colton in Chicago produced a very similar progestogen called norethynodrel – the main one used in the early contraceptive drug trials.

The stage was now set for the development of the pill as we know it. But many pharmaceutical companies feared the controversy that might result and were reluctant to apply these hormones for contraception, though they were happy for them to be used in the treatment of various gynaecological conditions. Margaret Sanger, with her wealthy friend Catherine McCormack, provided the encouragement and resources to researchers that eventually led to the marketing of the pill. The leaders of this work were the biologists Gregory Pincus and H. C. Chang, and the obstetrician John Rock. They worked first with animals and then used a small group of human volunteers in Boston. It soon became clear that the new hormones were very effective contraceptives, and produced no immediate or obvious harmful effects.

Trials with a larger number of women began in Puerto Rico in 1956, supervised by a young gynaecologist called Celso Ramón-Garcia and Edris Rice-Wray (the first female physician involved in testing the pill). The trials were highly successful – until, that is, the chemists got rid of an impurity in the pills. This impurity was the oestrogen, mestranol. Immediately things began to go wrong. Irregular bleeding occurred and so did accidental pregnancies. So it was really by chance that the researchers learnt that a little oestrogen was necessary for maximum effectiveness and control of the cycle. When they put it back in precise doses the combined pill was created. It took a few more years until June 1960 for the US Food and Drug Administration to release the first combination oestrogen and progestogen birth control pill Enovid-10. This contained what we would now consider far higher doses of the hormones than necessary.

35

It was agreed from the start that these new and powerful medicines should be distributed only under close supervision, and the initial recommendation was that they should not be used for more than two years continuously. They seemed to be safe but there was no certainty that they would prove to be so in the long term. Yet the pill was so much more acceptable than all previous methods of reversible family planning that women all over the world took to using it sooner and in greater numbers than almost anyone expected.

Mainland China, for example, has about 7 to 8 million current users. As well as pills, sheets of edible paper incorporating the hormones have been produced. These are stamped out into squares by perforations, just like a sheet of postage stamps. Each square can be labelled with a day of the week and taken daily in exactly the same way as ordinary pills. So far this does not appear to have caught on among Western manufacturers as an alternative to the usual tablets in 'blister' packs.

Figure 7 and Table 1 show the main ways by which the usual combined pill operates to prevent pregnancy. The main effect is to stop the normal hormone changes of the menstrual cycle and hence prevent both maturing of follicles and ovulation – (1) and (2) in the Table. However, there are several back-up mechanisms to make pregnancy unlikely even if egg-release should

Table 1 How combined pills prevent pregnancy
(The more +s means the greater the effect)

	'Ordinary' combined pills
1 Reduced FSH therefore follicles stopped from ripening and egg from maturing	++++
2 LH surge stopped so no egg-release	++++
3 Cervical mucus changed into a barrier to sperm	+++
4 Lining of uterus made less suitable for implantation of an embryo	+++
5 Uterine tubes perhaps affected so that they do not transport egg so well (uncertainty about this)	+
Expected pregnancy rate per 100 women using the pill method for one year (compare use of NO METHOD = 80–90)	0.1–1

Note: The combined pill is *very* reliable with plenty of back-up effects – but relies chiefly on effects 1 and 2. See Table 10 (page 182) for the progestogen-only pill.

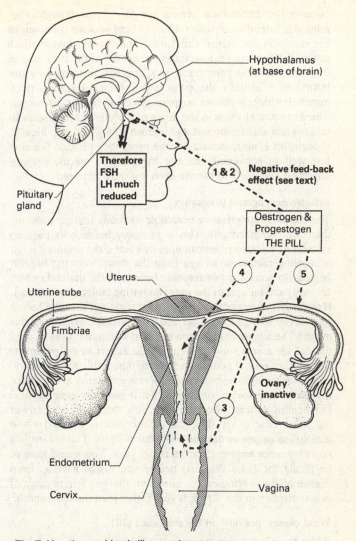

Fig. 7 How the combined pill prevents pregnancy

Note: Numbers 1–5 are the contraceptive effects of the combined pill as shown in Table 1

The following labels appear on the figure:

- Hypothalamus (at base of brain)
- **Therefore FSH LH much reduced**
- Pituitary gland
- **1 & 2** Negative feed-back effect (see text)
- Oestrogen & Progestogen THE PILL
- **4**
- **5**
- Uterus
- Uterine tube
- Fimbriae
- **3**
- Ovary inactive
- Endometrium
- Cervix
- Vagina

occur. (The commonest reason for this 'breakthrough' egg-release is forgetting to take tablets.) These back-up mechanisms are shown in the Figure and Table. The slippery mucus which normally flows from the cervix in the middle of the cycle and at that time is easily penetrated by sperm is transformed by the hormones – actually the progestogen – into a scanty, thick material which produces a quite effective barrier to sperm. There are also changes in the lining of the uterus which seem to make it less able to support and nourish a fertilized egg. Finally, though this is more debatable, the tubes may perhaps function less well in conveying the egg towards the uterus, perhaps making it less likely to survive even if it were fertilized.

Effectiveness against pregnancy

There is no more effective reversible method of family planning than the combined pill. This is probably because its back-up systems as just described can operate even if the prime effect of preventing release of an egg from the ovary were to fail. But failures do occur for two reasons: failures of the method (which are rare) and failures of the user (forgetting tablets: not so rare). If these two causes of failure are added together, the total failure rate can be as high as one per 100 woman-years. What does this mean? The simple explanation is that if a hundred women used the pill for a year, one of them should expect to get pregnant. Put another way, if you the user were to be fertile for 100 years, you would have an 'evens' chance of one pregnancy at the end of that time! Impossible, of course, but it gives the general idea. For healthy women who take their pills absolutely regularly at the same time every day, the failure rate is reduced about tenfold, to as low as 0.1 per 100 woman-years. This means just one pregnancy among 1,000 users per year. You would have to be fertile for 1,000 years (!) before you would have an even chance of one pregnancy . . . However, that one failure *could* of course happen in the very first year rather than the thousandth.

What causes 'periods' on the combined pill?

When the pill is taken the normal menstrual cycle is abolished. Just so long as sufficient of the artificial oestrogen and progestogen of the pill are in the bloodstream there will be no bleeding from the uterus. However, most women like to see some kind of period, as regular reassurance that the pill is working. It may also be better to reduce the monthly intake of artificial hormones to a minimum, and to give the pituitary and ovaries a break from time to time from the suppressing action of the pill hormones. For these reasons, and only for these reasons, most systems of pill-taking include a 6- or 7-day break every 28 days. The effect of thus cutting off the supply of pill hormones is

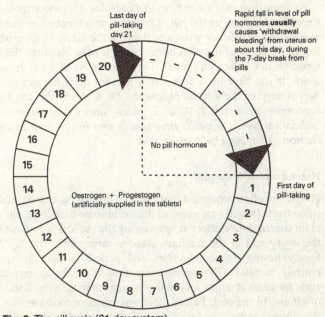

Fig. 8 The pill cycle (21-day system)
Note: Compare with Figure 6a. The normal cycle shown there is stopped and replaced by this simpler one which depends primarily on how the pill's hormones affect the uterus.

to *imitate* the fall in the levels in the bloodstream of their natural equivalents at the end of a normal cycle. This causes shedding of the rather thinner lining of the uterus which the pill's hormones have produced during the previous 21 days (see Figure 8). Because the lining is different – caused in a different way, by the pill, and looking different under the microscope – its shedding usually leads to less bleeding, often darker in colour, than a normal menstrual period. It is also a lot less likely to be painful.

So if you are on the pill your normal cycle is removed and replaced by something different. You are causing the 'periods' yourself by stopping the pills for one week out of every four. You could stop having periods altogether any time, if you in fact made no break from pill-taking. *As they are in reality substitute periods,* they are often more accurately called *hormone withdrawal bleeds*.

An important conclusion from all this is that if for some reason they fail to happen on the pill, it probably only means that there was too little artificially produced lining of the uterus that month for the stopping of the pill's hormones to lead to bleeding. 'Bad blood' is not 'piling up inside'. There just is *no blood to come away*. If you have been taking your pills regularly the explanation is very unlikely to be pregnancy. (If in doubt this can be confirmed by a test.) What is more, *absence of hormone withdrawal bleeds is totally irrelevant to any risk to your future chances of having a baby* (page 110).

How unnatural is the pill?

People are often concerned that even if it did not have unwanted side-effects (which I am going to discuss in some detail) the pill's main contraceptive effect in suppressing the cyclical activities of the ovary and of the pituitary gland is 'unnatural'. But is it? Surely having menstrual cycles and periods is actually not entirely 'natural'. Biologically, suppression of the menstrual cycle for years at a time may in fact be a much more natural state of affairs. In the past, before there was effective contraception, the normal thing was for a woman to be either pregnant or breast-feeding during all the child-bearing years. A doctor working in Central Africa once told me that he had been visited some years ago by a woman in her early forties who was worried by bleeding. By excluding all the other possibilities, he eventually diagnosed this as a normal period. She had been anxious because she never remembered having such a thing before!

Far from the myth that periods are normal and necessary to 'flush out the flues', they really are not what nature intends.

As support for this notion, it does seem that some cancers, such as cancer of the ovary, are commoner in women who have had more rather than less natural menstrual cycles during their lives. Probably for this reason, the pill seems to be protective against certain cancers (pages 122–3). Can we also be reassured by the fact that the pill's main action is to imitate the corpus luteum of pregnancy? Or that many of the changes in body chemistry caused by the pill (page 71), and not a few of the minor side-effects such as nausea, are so similar to those of pregnancy?

These questions cannot yet be given definite answers. Although in many ways the effects of the pill are similar to those of pregnancy, they are by no means all the same: and pregnancy is anyway not free of risks. What is more, the hormones used are artificial rather than natural. (So far, experiments using natural hormones in the pill have not been very satisfactory, but they are continuing.) The dosage of the two hormones is not exactly tailored to each individual. It is roughly constant for three weeks out of four rather than continuously varying as in the menstrual cycle. (So-called phased pills (page 168) imitate the menstrual cycle a little more closely, but still not perfectly.) And finally, the fact that some natural hormones are still produced by the woman's ovaries in addition to the artificial ones she is taking by mouth could have some effect.

So the most that should be said is that there are reasons to believe that the pill is not *quite* so unnatural as appears at first sight. In passing, it is a strange fact that some of the people who say the pill is 'unnatural' do something else which is equally unnatural, and on present evidence considerably more danger- ous – they smoke cigarettes! The pill contains two substances which are at least similar to hormones the body is used to handling. And pills are eaten – nothing in the animal kingdom takes food or alien chemicals on board through its lungs. The cigarette however is a chemical factory, manufacturing over 2,000 unnatural compounds *which are absorbed via the lungs to travel in the blood all over the body*. Some are known cancer-causing agents.

Research continues, and we certainly know a lot more now about the use of hormones for oral contraception than we did at the time of those early tests in Puerto Rico.

3
The pill: how do I
take it?

The progestogen-only pill (mini-pill) is considered in Chapter 8.

Systems of pill-taking

The most common system is the one in which you take *one pill daily for 21 days followed by a 7-day break*. There is one type of pill available in Britain and elsewhere which is taken for *22 days before a 6-day break*. Some women find this helpful, as the starting and finishing days are both on the same day of the week. In most countries other pill brands are available with 28 tablets in each packet, of which 7 are dummies, or 'blanks'. These are liked by many women. Care must be taken when starting these packets to avoid taking dummy pills at the wrong time, but the pills are taken consecutively, one packet after another. There is no need to remember when to stop and start taking successive courses. They have certain other advantages too (page 51.)

There is another way to take pills, called the *three-monthly or 'tricycle' system*. In this, four packets are taken in succession – therefore a pill every day for 84 days – followed by a 6- or 7-day break during which the three-monthly 'period' normally occurs. As explained in the last chapter, pill 'periods' are in fact 'hormone withdrawal bleeds', created artificially by the taking of a 7-day break. So there is no particular reason why they should happen every four weeks. Once this has been explained, many women have found this four-periods-per-year routine quite acceptable, indeed preferable. A word of caution though: it is a fact that you will have taken one-third more of the artificial hormones in each three months than you would following the more usual system of pill-taking. This might tend to increase the risk of some side-effects (page 131). Some doctors, myself among them, are therefore not entirely happy about this tricycle scheme, unless there is a special reason (headaches for example, which can be an excellent reason, see pages 96–7).

The tricycle system of pill-taking is of course completely different from triphasic pills, which are described on page 168.

Postponing 'periods'

Even if you regularly use the three weeks on, one week off system, one advantage of the pill is that there is no objection on special occasions to your postponing your 'periods'. This can be done either by taking extra pills from a spare packet, or more simply by just taking two packets in succession. Some women do this initially in order to avoid ever having bleeding at weekends; or subsequently on special occasions such as a holiday. Note, however, that there are special rules for phased pills (pages 170–1) and that it is *not* recommended that you bring your 'period' on sooner by stopping pill-taking early. This might lead to a pregnancy.

Whenever you take the *7-day break* from pill-taking, your protection against pregnancy continues throughout it, provided three things are true:

(a) you have been regular in your pill-taking from the preceding packet;

(b) none of the other conditions which might reduce your protection has applied in your case (see pages 49–59);

(c) you do in fact start another packet on the eighth day.

If (c) is not true, sperm might perhaps survive so long inside the uterus that if they arrived there after love-making on the sixth or seventh day after the last pill, they *might* be able to fertilize any egg released and entering the uterine tube early in the following week.

How to start taking the pill

If you are having normal periods up to the time of starting the pill, there are two ways to start. *The standard method* is to take the first pill on the fifth day of your period, whether your bleeding has stopped or not. Choose a pill from the section on the packet marked with that day of the week and press down on

43

the plastic bubble so as to remove it from the foil on the reverse side. Then take a pill a day for 21 days (22 days for some brands). After a 7-day break you then start taking pills again on the eighth day: and from then on in each four weeks you follow the regular routine of 21 days of pill-taking followed by a 7-day break. (Avoid making a common mistake here, which is to start each new packet like the first on the fifth day of the period. This can cause a pregnancy, if the 'period' happens to come on late.)

An example of a diary card kept by a woman using this method is shown in Figure 9. Notice that she started her first packet on 14 May, the fifth day of her period, while she was still bleeding; but subsequent pill 'periods' in June and July were shorter and lighter and occurred during each 7-day break from taking pills. Note too that there is a 7-day break between packets whenever the 'period' occurs (or even if it fails to appear). So the fifth-day-of-the-period rule only applies to the very first packet.

The snag of this system is that some women frequently and others quite unexpectedly can have short menstrual cycles. There is then the risk that by the fifth day of the first course of pills, there may already be a follicle ripening. This could be producing so much natural oestrogen that the pill may be unable to stop the surge of LH hormone from the pituitary which leads to release of an egg (see page 29 and Figures 4 and 5). And so it is generally recommended that until the 14th pill of the first course has been taken (which is the same thing as the eighteenth day from the start of that first period) you should use an effective alternative method of family planning as well, such as the sheath. These 'unsafe days' are shown in Figure 9 by an × in the Remarks section. Obviously it is a bit of a nuisance to be unable to rely on the pill straight away.

Starting on the first day of the period

If, in the first cycle only of pill-taking, you start the tablets on the very first day of the period, egg-release is effectively prevented even among women with short cycles. Thus no extra method of family planning need be used. The only problem is that in the first pill cycle this method does seem to cause a bit more 'breakthrough bleeding' which is bleeding on days when you are taking tablets. A part of this is only to be expected, during the first few days, when you are deliberately taking pills during the

44

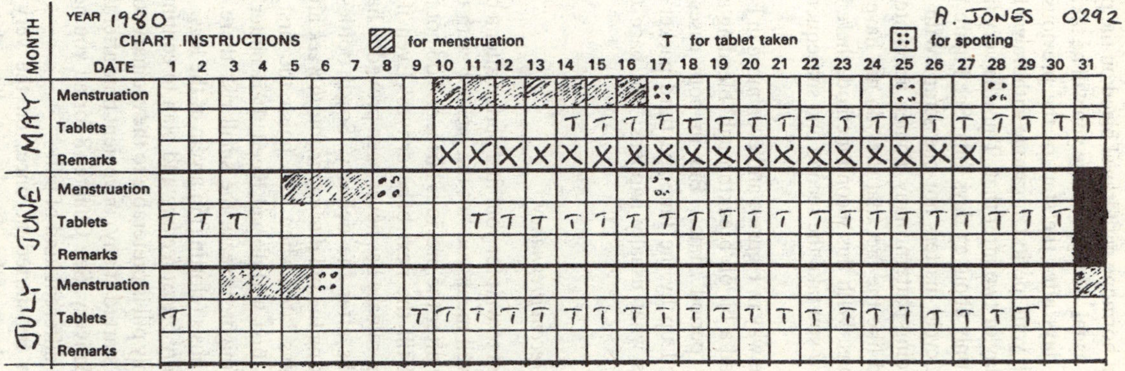

Fig. 9 Diary card – 5th day start of the pill

Note: X in remarks = reminder that the sheath should be used if any intercourse before the 14th pill is taken.

YEAR 1980

A. JONES 0292

CHART INSTRUCTIONS

⬛ for menstruation T for tablet taken ⬚ for spotting

MONTH		DATE	1	2	3	4	5	6	7	8	9	10	11	12	13	14	15	16	17	18	19	20	21	22	23	24	25	26	27	28	29	30	31
MAY		Menstruation																															
		Tablets	T	T	T												T	T	T	T	T	T	T	T	T	T	T	T	T	T	T	T	T
		Remarks																				X	X	X	X	X	X	X	X				
JUNE		Menstruation																															
		Tablets			T	T										T	T	T	T	T	T	T	T	T	T	T	T	T	T	T	T	T	
		Remarks										X	X	X	X	X	X	X															
JULY		Menstruation																															
		Tablets	T									T	T	T	T	T	T	T	T	T	T	T	T	T	T	T	T	T	T	T	T		
		Remarks																															

45

bleeding of that first period. Another important point to realize is that your first hormone withdrawal bleed on the pill will come on sooner than usual. This is because you will be taking your 21st tablet only 21 days after the start of the previous period. As usual on the pill your 'period'/hormone withdrawal bleeding will follow only a day or two after that. Thus the very first pill cycle will tend to be only about 23 days long. See Figure 10.

A short first cycle matters not one scrap. With forewarning about the bleeding pattern many women are quite happy with this system and like the fact that they do not have to take any extra precautions. With this second method, there is no change of course in how you take the second and subsequent packets of pills.

Notice by the way in Figure 9 and even more in Figure 10 that both women had a bit of 'breakthrough' bleeding and spotting, other than at 'period' times. But in both cases this minor problem cleared up by the time the third packet of pills was started. This is what usually happens. See page 60 for more about this.

Starting after a recent pregnancy

There is no need to wait for your first period after a baby. Indeed to do so may well mean you 'hit the jackpot' with the very first egg you release after the previous birth, and do not therefore see another period till the next babe arrives! Even if you do not breast-feed, egg-release has never been proved to happen earlier than four weeks after the delivery. So, if bottle-feeding you should start taking the pill *during the fourth week* after the birth. Twenty-one days later when you finish the first packet you should see the first withdrawal bleed. It is better not to start earlier as this might increase the small risk there is, after any birth, of thrombosis (clotting) in a vein of the legs.

If you are *fully breast-feeding* and plan to continue, then the progestogen-only pill is preferable to the ordinary combined pill. This pill can be started at any convenient time after the first week following the delivery. See Chapter 8 for all you need to know about this very different kind of pill.

The pill can be started at once, on the very day of the procedure – or the next day if you are feeling a bit sick – after a

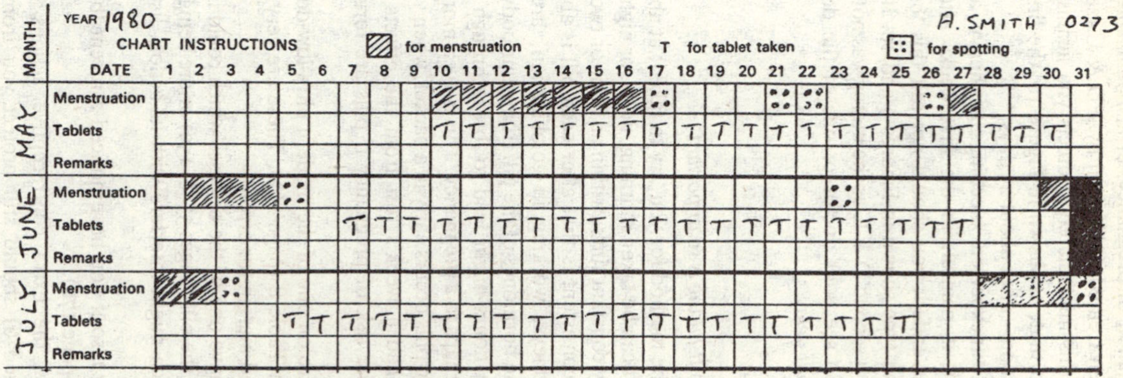

Fig. 10 Diary card – 1st day start of the pill

suction termination of pregnancy, or a *spontaneous miscarriage* which has been treated in hospital by a D & C (see Glossary). Starting like this immediately protects you against pregnancy, and will mean that, as shown in Figure 10, the first period will occur rather soon – after about 23 days.

If you get unexpected bleeding, as heavy as a period, especially if it is painful, in the first weeks after any early pregnancy has ended, you should *not* call this 'breakthrough' bleeding of the type shown in Figures 9 and 10. It could mean that you need a second D & C as the uterus was not emptied out completely. So see your doctor or one of the doctors at the hospital *without delay*.

Why regular pill-taking is so important

If the pill is the method for you, try to take it at about the same time of day. It can be taken morning, noon, or night as long as it is at a roughly constant time, within an hour or two. The reason for being so consistent is that after each pill is absorbed, your liver and kidneys, working in combination, are continually eliminating the hormones of the pill from your body. So a gap of more than 24 hours *might* lead to 'breakthrough' egg-release: and hence perhaps to a pregnancy. This is even more likely if the delay in taking pills occurs early in a packet, when your body has anyway just had a week's rest from the effects of the pill's hormones. The risk of pregnancy if pills are forgotten is also greater:

(a) if you are on one of the modern ultra-low-dose combined pills shown in Table 8 (page 162). These are very reliable, but have a reduced margin for error;

(b) if you have one of the diseases which could interfere with absorption of the pill (pages 53–6, 159) or are being treated with any drug which might interfere with its action, listed on pages 56–8;

(c) possibly also if you have noticed a recent 'breakthrough' bleeding (see page 176).

Fortunately, the extra contraceptive actions described in Table 1 (page 36) should still protect you from pregnancy, especially if you obey the rules which follow.

Circumstances which may reduce protection against pregnancy

Missed pills

Do not panic if you forget to take a pill. This is one of the commonest worries that any pill-user ever has. It is unlikely that you will become pregnant. However, it is certainly not something to make a habit of, and most pregnancies on the pill are caused this way. To be as safe as can be you need to follow some simple rules. You will find it helpful throughout this section to keep referring to Figure 11.

If you have remembered within less than 12 hours, for instance next morning if you usually take the pill at night, all you need to do is to take the forgotten pill immediately and then return to your daily routine, taking your next pill at the usual time, even if this means taking two on the same day. If the delay is more than 12 hours take the omitted pill and the next one at the usual time, and then complete the course followed by the 7-day break as usual: but consider yourself no longer sufficiently protected by the pill for the next 14 days. In other words, *for the next 14 days use another effective method as well as the pill whatever happens,* continuing if need be during the early days of pill-taking from the next packet. Disregard for this purpose any bleeding that occurs. If it is the unexpected 'breakthrough' type on pill-taking days, keep taking the pills. If it is your expected bleeding during the pill-free week, keep on using the other method – unless and until the 14 days are up. THIS IS THE 14-DAY RULE.

What is another effective method? Whenever another method is mentioned and any type of pill has recently been or is being taken, this must never be the rhythm, temperature, or cervical mucus methods. The pill's hormones make these quite unusable. Family planners do not recommend spermicides used alone either, and the intra-uterine device (IUD) or coil is unlikely to be useful for so short a time. So what is really meant is either abstinence or a barrier method such as the sheath or one of the types of cap such as the diaphragm used with a spermicide (see page 222).

The rules here and in Figure 11 are likely to be different from the rules in the leaflet with your packet of pills, and these often differ from one manufacturer to another. However they are the same as in the leaflets issued by the British Family Planning

49

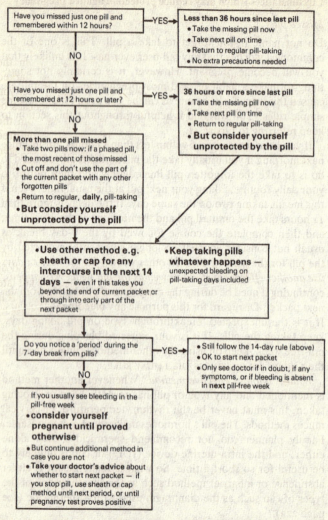

Have you missed just one pill and remembered within 12 hours? —YES→ **Less than 36 hours since last pill**
- Take the missing pill now
- Take next pill on time
- Return to regular pill-taking
- No extra precautions needed

↓ NO

Have you missed just one pill and remembered at 12 hours or later? —YES→ **36 hours or more since last pill**
- Take the missing pill now
- Take next pill on time
- Return to regular pill-taking
- **But consider yourself unprotected by the pill**

↓ NO

More than one pill missed
- Take two pills now: if a phased pill, the most recent of those missed
- Cut off and don't use the part of the current packet with any other forgotten pills
- Return to regular, **daily**, pill-taking
- **But consider yourself unprotected by the pill**

- **Use other method e.g. sheath or cap for any intercourse in the next 14 days** — even if this takes you beyond the end of current packet or through into early part of the next packet

- **Keep taking pills whatever happens** — unexpected bleeding on pill-taking days included

Do you notice a 'period' during the 7-day break from pills? —YES→
- Still follow the 14-day rule (above)
- OK to start next packet
- Only see doctor if in doubt, if any symptoms, or if bleeding is absent in **next** pill-free week

↓ NO

If you usually see bleeding in the pill-free week
- **consider yourself pregnant until proved otherwise**
- But continue additional method in case you are not
- Take your doctor's advice about whether to start next packet — if you stop pill, use sheath or cap method until next period, or until pregnancy test proves positive

Fig. 11 What to do when pills are taken late or missed altogether

Note: For progestogen-only pill see Figure 18 (pages 188–9).

Association. What is the justification for this 14-day rule?

In all women the menstrual cycle is taken away during the 21 days of pill-taking. But during the pill-free week we have demonstrated at the Margaret Pyke Centre that the blood levels of FSH (from the pituitary gland) and oestrogen (from the ovaries) tend to rise. In some women the rise is more marked than others. If you understood pages 30–3 of the last chapter you will realize that this suggests that the pituitary and ovaries of these women are, if you like, struggling to get free from the suppressing effect of the pill. Any lengthening of the pill-free time beyond seven days means a risk that the level of oestrogen will get to a high enough level in a few women at least, to cause a 'surge' of LH and hence egg-release from the largest follicle (see page 32). And egg-release means the risk of pregnancy.

How could the pill-free time be lengthened?

One obvious way is by *forgetting one or more pills at the beginning of a packet.* In fact these are about the most important of all pills to remember to take. Going away for a weekend or longer without one's pills and hence starting the next packet late is a well-known cause of unplanned pregnancy in pill-takers. It is one reason why I personally favour the more widespread use of 28-day pill packaging as described on page 42. (A woman who is used to taking pills all the time is less likely to forget to take her packet wherever she goes.)

The rule should protect a woman who misses out pills early in a packet. She must not rely on the pill method for 14 days from the moment she discovers the problem. The first week of this time is the time of greatest pregnancy risk, and there is no need to continue with precautions right to the end of the packet, if this means more than 14 days.

How else might the pill-free time be lengthened?

Another way would be by *missing pills at the end of the previous packet,* and then still taking the usual 7-day break. In this case the dangerous time for conceiving would not be when the pills were forgotten, but over a week later when – once again – the pituitary and ovary have been 'let off the hook' for longer than usual. In other words they will have had more than the usual time in which to get ready for egg-release. The same rule should be followed, but here the more 'dangerous' time is the *second week* of the 14 days.

Interestingly, in this situation – pills missed out at end of the previous packet – pregnancy could result from intercourse during or after the withdrawal bleeding. This is because that bleeding is not truly a period (page 38–9), being caused only by the earlier withdrawal of the artificial hormones. It has no connection with what is happening at the ovary. The egg could be released any time around the end of the pill-free week *if it has been made longer than a week by pills missed at the end of the previous packet.*

What about missing pills in the middle of a packet?

Contrary to what most pill-takers – and some doctors – think, this is the least dangerous time to miss pills. If you follow the argument here, you will see that egg-release and pregnancy are less likely because the pills are missed after the pituitary and ovary have been 'quietened' by several days of pill-taking. All the same you would still be safer if you did not rely on the pill method for 14 days. This is indeed recommended *whenever* in the packet a pill is taken more than 12 hours late.

What if I have been so disorganized that I forgot a succession of pills?

To take a handful of pills will simply make you sick! Take two pills at once: this still might make you feel a bit queasy but does help to reduce the chance of your becoming pregnant. If you are taking a phased pill, (page 168) the two pills you swallow should be the *most recent* of those missed. You should push out and discard any other forgotten pills. This will ensure that the next tablet, which should follow at the next regular time, will correspond with the correct day of the week as marked on your packet. You should consider yourself completely unprotected by the pill for the next 14 days and also at some risk of having conceived if you had intercourse during the time before you woke up to the fact that you were not taking the pills. All is not lost, however, and here you should follow most faithfully the rules shown in Figure 11. You should also read the answers to the next two questions very carefully, particularly the one 'What if my next "period" does not come on?'

What else may happen? Even if egg-release does not occur as a result of omitted pills, you are also now more likely to get the problem of *'breakthrough' bleeding*.

This is a spotting or sometimes a rather heavier loss, coming on at any time other than the pill-free week. It happens for the same reason as the normal pill 'period': too little of the effect of the pill's hormones reaching the lining of the uterus. However, it will almost always stop if you simply disregard it and take pills regularly from now on, using the usual 21 days on, 7 days off routine.

What if my next 'period' does not come on? In brief, take advice from your doctor, but continue using some other safe method of family planning like the sheath. This is advisable because absent withdrawal bleeding is only rarely due to pregnancy (see page 40). It would be a pity to become unnecessarily pregnant because you thought you already were, so to speak! Taking the pill will not stop the pregnancy test becoming positive. If new symptoms like nausea, or having to pass urine very frequently, occur – even if you have taken your pills regularly in fact – you should see your doctor in case they might be due to pregnancy. Take with you for testing a small amount of your first urine of the day in a clean container.

Taking the pill in early pregnancy has not been proved to harm babies (page 110). All the same if you do strongly suspect that you might be pregnant as a result of a pill-taking muddle, most doctors recommend that you transfer to using something like the sheath method, carefully, until you know one way or another. This would also normally be the best policy if for any reason you were unable to discuss the matter with a doctor.

But if you have absolutely *no* reason to suspect reduced protection, then it is in my view best to start the next packet even if there is no bleeding in the pill-free week. It would be necessary to see your doctor and arrange a pregnancy test if you began getting the symptoms of pregnancy, or if you went on to miss a second period. See also pages 176–7.

Stomach upsets

From the body's point of view these mean the same as forgetting to take the pills, so the risk of 'breakthrough' egg-release and of

● Diarrhoea

● Vomiting

Did you vomit more than 3 hours after taking a pill?

NO

Less than 3 hours
• Take a further pill (from end of packet, or a separate one)

Does the second pill stay down? and:
Was it taken less than 12 hours after your regular time for pill-taking?

NO

• Get back to regular pill-taking as soon as you can keep pills down
• **But consider yourself unprotected by the pill from the first day of vomiting**

YES

• Take next pill on time
• Return to regular pill-taking
• No extra precautions needed

Did loose bowel actions start more than 12 hours after the last pill and finish by the time of the next one, with no recurrence?

YES

• No action required
• Continue regular pill-taking

NO

• Continue regular pill-taking
• **But consider yourself unprotected by the pill from the first day of diarrhoea**

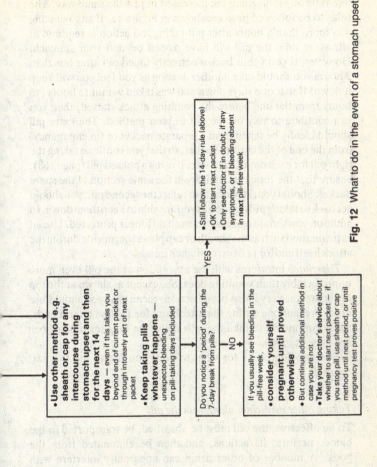

- **Use other method e.g. sheath or cap for any intercourse during stomach upset and then for the next 14 days** — even if this takes you beyond end of current packet or through into early part of next packet
- **Keep taking pills whatever happens** — unexpected bleeding on pill-taking days included

Do you notice a 'period' during the 7-day break from pills?

YES →
- Still follow the 14-day rule (above)
- OK to start next packet
- Only see doctor if in doubt, if any symptoms, or if bleeding absent in **next pill-free week**

NO
If you usually see bleeding in the pill-free week,
- **consider yourself pregnant until proved otherwise**
- But continue additional method in case you are not
- **Take your doctor's advice about** whether to start next packet — if you stop pill, use sheath or cap method until next period, or until pregnancy test proves positive

Fig. 12 What to do in the event of a stomach upset

55

'breakthrough' bleeding are increased in just the same way. The rules to be followed here are shown in Figure 12. If any *vomiting* was more than 3 hours after pill-taking, no action is required at all, as by then the pill will have passed beyond your stomach. However, if you vomit back a correctly timed pill after less than 3 hours you should take another as soon as you feel you will keep it down. If that one stays down and was taken within 12 hours (36 hours from the one before the vomiting attack started) then you can continue to rely on the pill as your method. The extra pill should ideally be taken from a separate packet or (in emergency) from the end of the current packet, so that you continue taking the right pill for each day of the week. If using a phased pill (page 168), ensure that the replacement is from the same section of the spare packet. Should your stomach also reject the second pill, you should get back to taking pills as soon as you are able to keep them down. In addition you should consider yourself no longer protected. Use an extra method such as the sheath or cap plus a spermicide during the attack itself and for 14 days from when it ends.

Diarrhoea interferes with the absorption of the pill even more unpredictably than vomiting does. So, except as shown at the top of Figure 12, very loose bowel actions mean that you should use other precautions during the attack and for 14 days after it ends, while continuing to take the pills daily. On long-term diarrhoea see pages 159–60.

See also Figure 11 for what to do if you fail to see the next 'period'.

Taking other medicines along with the pill

To be effective, the pill must be absorbed, be transported in the blood, perform its actions, and then be eliminated from the body. A number of other drugs can apparently interfere with some of these complex processes. Such interference (interaction) can lower the blood levels of the pill hormones and so lead to the risk of egg-release and therefore pregnancy. See Table 2a.

This effect can be caused in various ways, including a stimulating action on the special liver enzymes which normally inactivate the hormones before they are disposed of in the urine. There is the possibility too that some antibiotics might interfere with the absorption of oestrogen hormone from the gut, or with

56

the special system there is for re-absorbing any which subsequently escapes back there from the liver via the bile. (This antibiotic effect does not affect progestogen and therefore causes no problem for users of the POP – page 186.)

Women on long-term treatment with a relevant drug, especially for tuberculosis or epilepsy, may have to consider another method altogether. After discussion though, many can continue to use the pill under careful medical supervision. They should naturally use a slightly higher-dose pill from the list in Table 9 (page 163) rather than an ultra-low-dose pill (Table 8, page 162). Following the reasoning on pages 49–52, it might also be advised that they take a shorter break than usual between pill packets – e.g. just 5 days. This should reduce the risk of egg-release.

The golden rules are obviously:

(a) to tell the person who prescribes you the pill about all other drugs you are taking, and

(b) to inform any other doctor about to prescribe you any drug that you use the pill. During and for 14 days after a short course of antibiotics, for *maximum* security use an extra contraceptive. This seems unnecessary if you take long-term low-dose tetra-cycline for acne, except preferably at the start of treatment. Extra oestrogen (i.e. a Table 9 pill) will further reduce the pregnancy risk – and improve the acne. See page 179.

The risk must be very small as ampicillin (Penbritin), which is one of the common antibiotics that have been blamed for causing this problem, has often been given to pill-users without any pregnancies resulting. Recent research suggests that it is only a very small minority of women whose blood levels of the pill hormones are markedly lowered by ampicillin treatment.

Watch for 'breakthrough' bleeding (see page 176 for more details). Even if the other drug you are taking, perhaps one you bought yourself at the chemist, is not on the list in Table 2a – but particularly if it is – watch out for bleeding on tablet-taking days. This so-called 'breakthrough' bleeding coming on for the first time after starting another drug can be *the early warning sign of too low a blood level of the pill's hormones,* and hence an increased chance of pregnancy. It should always make you discuss the matter promptly with whoever prescribed you the pill. And use an additional method like the sheath until advised that it is no longer necessary.

57

Table 2a Drugs which are suspected of interfering with the pill, to cause 'breakthrough' bleeding and increased risk of pregnancy. Evidence for this is stronger for some drugs on this list (in *italic*) than for others. Common brand names are in brackets.

Drugs to treat epilepsy

phenobarbitone (Luminal)	*ethosuximide (Zarontin)*
and other barbiturates	*primidone (Mysoline)*
phenytoin (Epanutin)	*carbamazepine (Tegretol)*

The only drugs for epilepsy that do not interfere appear to be sodium valproate (Epilim) and clonazepam (Rivotril). But these are not necessarily the right choice.

Sedatives and tranquillizers

chlorpromazine (Largactil)	meprobamate (Equanil)

Drugs to treat infections

rifampicin (Rimactane) – used in the treatment of *tuberculosis*
Many other antibiotics, such as *ampicillin (Penbritin)* and *tetracyclines*, are also under suspicion of interfering with the combined pill only, not POP – but see note below.

Miscellaneous drugs

spironolactone (Aldactone)	dichloralphenazone (Welldorm)
griseofulvin (Grisovin)	glutethimide (Doriden)
phenylbutazone (Butazolidin)	

Cigarette smoke

There is surprising new evidence that smoking *may* reduce the pill's contraceptive effects

---

Note: **This is *not* a complete list.** Other drug interactions remain to be discovered. Several have been deliberately omitted because so far there is too little evidence that, in practice, they cause any problem for pill-users. Co-trimoxazole (Septrin), and possibly metronidazole (Flagyl), actually enhance the pill's effects – like Vitamin C (page 76), though not for the same reason.

Effect of the pill on other drugs

The opposite kind of interference is also possible, in which the pill alters the action of another drug. Table 2b gives one or two known examples. This whole problem of drugs interfering with each other highlights the tendency these days to take too many medicines of all kinds, maybe sometimes without a very good reason.

If in doubt about any kind of drug interaction or whether or not you may rely on the pill alone, ASK YOUR DOCTOR.

Change of pills from a higher- to a lower- or ultra-low-dose variety

This matter of the different brands of pills will make more sense when you have read Chapter 7. However, the question of changing to a lower-dose pill needs to be considered here, as this is another time when there could be some loss of contraceptive

58

✳ Table 2b Interference in the opposite direction: i.e. it is suspected that the pill may alter the effects of the other drug

---

Drugs to treat diabetes

The dose of insulin or oral tablet treatments may sometimes need to be increased. This is rarely a problem, and diabetics are *usually* advised to use other contraceptive methods anyway (page 156).

Some drugs for treating depression/anxiety or immune disorders

Their effectiveness may be altered by the pill. Also reported: a slightly increased chance of toxic effects of the other drug.

chlordiazepoxide (Librium)	diazepam (Valium)	imipramine (Tofranil)
amitriptyline (Tryptizol)	prednisolone (Prednesol)	

Drugs for treating high blood pressure

The effectiveness of the drug in lowering blood pressure may be reduced (but the pill is best avoided anyway – page 156).

Migraine treatments containing

ergotamine (Cafergot, Migril)   dihydroergotamine (Dihydergot)

If these drugs, which act by narrowing down the arteries, are taken by a pill-user, there may be an increase in the otherwise very small risk of arterial thrombosis (pages 80–5).

Anti-coagulants

warfarin – variably affected, anti-clotting effect becomes difficult to control. Should not normally be used by pill-takers.

---

protection. At the change-over time the steady suppression by the pill of the woman's natural hormones from her pituitary and ovary is reduced, just enough perhaps to allow 'breakthrough' egg-release. However, once she is safely established on the new low- or ultra-low-dose pill, she is effectively protected against pregnancy. The extra pregnancy risk is only at the time of the change-over and is small. It can be virtually eliminated by taking extra precautions for two weeks if there is the usual gap between packets; or more simply, by *starting the new lower-dose variety the very next day after finishing the current higher-dose packet*. Pills are then taken daily for 21 days, followed by a 7-day break recommencing on the eighth day for a further 21 days and so on as usual.

If you follow this system you may have bleeding like a pill 'period' during the first 7 days of tablet-taking from your new low-dose packet. Or you may have no bleeding at all till after the end of that new packet. Either is quite normal, and your protection against pregnancy is maintained throughout.

This problem never of course arises when moving to a higher-dose pill, which can be done after the usual 7-day break. For the rules about changing from a combined (ordinary) pill to a progestogen-only variety or back again, see Chapter 8.

Side-effects

These are all going to be considered fully later, but a few general points need making here in this practical chapter about pill-taking.

Side-effects are effects extra to the main actions of any drug which in the case of the pill are those shown in Table 1 (page 36). They can be good or bad, and the good ones are much too often forgotten. The effects which are unwanted fall into two main types: *uncommon side-effects*, some of which can be serious; and *commoner* ones which are almost never serious but do cause enough nuisance or trouble to make some people change to a different pill or perhaps a different method.

Considering the commoner ones first, they can be divided into two further groups as follows:

1. *Side-effects related to the bleeding pattern*

● *'Breakthrough' bleeding and spotting* (bleeding or spotting on tablet-taking days)

● *Absence of pill 'periods'* (no bleeding on the tablet-free days) See page 53.

More details about how these problems can be handled are given in Chapter 7 along with a helpful diagram (Figure 17, pages 174–5).

Except on the advice of your doctor, *neither* problem should be allowed to affect your daily pill-taking routine. Let the pill packet rule your pill-taking, not the bleeding pattern – whatever that may be. Do not stop taking pills before the end of a packet because of bleeding even if it seems like a period. Pregnancies have happened that way . . . Just keep taking successive packets and wait for the arrival of the normal bleeding pattern in due course. If in doubt, see your doctor: especially if reduced protection is a possibility (pages 49–59).

2. *Other so-called minor side-effects*

These include nausea, headaches, breast tenderness or tingling, gain in weight, vaginal discharge, leg aches and cramps, mild depression, and loss of interest in sex. All these and more have been reported by pill-users, but don't cross bridges. You may well have no side-effects at all and could even feel extra well while taking the pill. This is much more commonly so now that the dose given has been so much reduced. However, every woman reacts in her own special way, and the first pill tried is not always the best for you. As there are more than 20 varieties of pill, if you do have problems, it is usually possible to find a different brand that suits you better. This is all fully discussed using the idea of 'pill ladders' in Chapter 7 (Figures 15–17, pages 161–80).

A very important point to remember is to give any particular brand a good try before giving up, and this usually means using it for at least three months. If either bleeding or other-type minor side-effects occur, they usually do settle down after the first two or three courses of pills. If you look again at the list above, several of the symptoms, such as nausea, breast tenderness, and gain in weight, also happen in the first few months of pregnancy. This is partly because the pill imitates pregnancy in some ways, but it is probably just a coincidence that, as in pregnancy, the symptoms usually improve after the third month!

More major or serious side-effects

These are also discussed in much more detail later. For completeness I am including here a list of those symptoms which, though most unlikely to occur, should lead you to contact a doctor at once and to inform him or her that you are taking the pill. They may or may not mean anything serious or even be anything to do with the pill. *But they do mean that you should*

(a) *stop the pill until further notice* (but transfer to using another effective method)

(b) *come under medical care without delay*

so the diagnosis can be made and the right treatment started.

1. Severe pain in the calf of one leg, especially if linked with swelling (not the aching legs that so many people get, nor simple painless swelling of both ankles).

2. Severe central pain in the chest. Severe sharp pains in either side of the chest, aggravated by breathing.

3. Unexplained breathlessness, or cough with blood-stained phlegm.

4. Severe pain in the abdomen.

5. Any unusually severe, prolonged headache, particularly if of migraine type, especially if it is the first ever such attack or gets worse with the passage of time or keeps returning.

6. A bad fainting attack or collapse.

7. Sudden weakness, or *very marked* numbness and tingling *suddenly* affecting one side or one part of the body. NB This is not to be confused with the carpal tunnel syndrome, page 118.

8. Sudden loss of part of the field of vision.

9. Sudden disturbance of the ability to speak normally.

10. A severe and generalized, perhaps painful, skin rash (page 117).

11. Jaundice (yellow eyes and skin).

12. Very high blood pressure (page 150).

Number 12 is something which can be diagnosed by a doctor or nurse only when routinely measuring the blood pressure. Also jaundice may well first be noticed by a doctor or other observer.

These are practically the only reasons important enough for the pill to be stopped at once, in the middle of a packet. Otherwise make a routine appointment to see your doctor and continue to the end of a packet. This reduces the chance of an unplanned pregnancy (and erratic bleeding). In fact if the doctor is able to reassure you that your symptom from the list above is not due to anything serious and *not* due to the pill, you can of course restart pill-taking, following the rules of Figure 11.

Just because you see a frightening list of symptoms like the one here does not mean that you will ever experience a single one of them. Indeed, this is most unlikely.

Two other reasons for stopping the pill

1. *Immobilization*. This means being confined to bed, as might occur rather suddenly, for instance after an accident. It is recommended that you stop the pill at once as being kept in bed makes blood clotting in the veins of the leg more probable, and the pill may increase that risk.

2. *Major operations*. The chances of a blood clot in deep veins of the legs are increased by the operation itself, as well as by the confinement to bed which obviously follows it. Being on the pill will of course never stop you having an emergency, life-saving, operation such as for appendicitis. However, if a fairly big operation such as removal of your gall-bladder is planned, it is sensible to stop taking the pill *six weeks beforehand* and for at least four weeks afterwards. From the time you stop the pill to going into hospital for your operation it is of course most important to use some other effective family planning method.

Unless your gynaecologist tells you otherwise, it is usually perfectly in order for you to continue on the pill right up to the time of a female sterilization procedure – which is a minor operation – and then just to finish the current packet.

Coming off the pill

There is no need to make any routine breaks from the pill every few months or years in order to preserve your fertility or for any other reason. Secondly, after stopping the pill it is very common for the first spontaneous or natural period to be a bit delayed. But two-thirds of women have their first period by six weeks after their last pill 'period', and by six months nearly all have got back their own periods. So a 'wait and see' policy is best. If this, or anything else, is a worry to you do not hesitate to discuss it with your family doctor or with the clinic doctor who prescribes you the pill. Actually, many women find out the hard way that their fertility is in fine shape after stopping the pill: by getting pregnant so very easily that they cannot believe it! So if you are not ready for a baby, be warned and use another safe method from the day you stop. N.B. *Not the rhythm method* – this is totally unreliable following a course of pills. See pages 221–3.

If you go overdue after stopping the pill you may be worried that your new method of family planning has let you down. In that case wait until it is at least six weeks since your last pill 'period', which is four weeks from the earliest likely egg-release. Then arrange a pregnancy test on a small amount of your first urine of the day. Commonly it will be negative and remain so if repeated, until you see your first natural period in due course.

Very occasionally the first period is very much delayed, and if so it is sensible to take medical advice: but not until six months have gone by. A few tests are essential, to check that your pituitary gland and ovaries are in good working order, though currently 'resting'. But usually nothing more needs to be done to bring back your menstrual cycle, with the usual release of eggs and periods: until, that is, you wish to try for a baby.

Stopping the pill to have a baby

Obstetricians much prefer that women who stop the pill for this reason use another contraceptive method, such as the sheath or the diaphragm, until they have seen at least one natural period – which means one later than the bleeding which followed a few days after the last packet of pills. This helps them to calculate the date the baby is due. Some experts think that *ideally* you should wait for three months as well as for one period, before trying for a baby. See page 110. There is no proof yet that this is beneficial, though it can do no harm.

The 'morning after' pill – post-coital contraception

Despite the name, it is possible to use hormone treatment to prevent pregnancy starting a bit later than the next morning after unprotected intercourse – up to 72 hours later in fact. Accidents do happen – sheaths rupturing or slipping off, for instance; not to mention rape. In my view there are therefore definitely some cases for whom this treatment is appropriate. It is believed to act by preventing implantation (page 29), so it is not causing an abortion. Others may disagree: see page 206 for discussion of some ethical aspects.

Nowadays the usual hormone treatment is two tablets of a particular 50 mcg oestrogen-containing pill, taken in the doctor's surgery or clinic, followed by two more exactly twelve hours later. You will notice that I do not name the pill brand(s) used. This is deliberate. Readers should resist the temptation to 'dabble' in this kind of treatment, without medical supervision.

Why a doctor should be involved

Correct use of the correct pills is important. A vaginal examination and blood pressure check should be done before treatment and subsequent to the next period. Side-effects occur, chiefly nausea, sometimes vomiting. Even the decision to treat at all is not that simple. In some cases there could be reasons for withholding the treatment. The chances of conception can sometimes be judged by the doctor to be so low that the risks of treatment are greater than those of just waiting for the next period. The other type of treatment, with an IUD (page 204) put in up to five days after ovulation, may occasionally be medically preferable: for instance because the hormone method is less effective beyond 72 hours after intercourse, or if other risks were also taken earlier in the cycle. If there is already a pregnancy the

64

hormone treatment will not cause an abortion. The method can fail, in about two in a hundred cases treated. And the possibility of a pregnancy being harmed by the hormones cannot be ruled out, though the risk is thought to be *less* than the estimate on page 113. Very rarely, an ectopic pregnancy can occur, page 192.

All in all this 'morning after' treatment is not that simple and should be used only in emergency, not repeatedly as a method of birth control. The need for it should be removed by arranging a recognized method for the future. As the hormone method can sometimes work by just delaying egg-release, it is important to use a method like the sheath until the start of the next period anyway. In appropriate cases, insertion of an IUD has the obvious advantage of solving both the immediate and the longer-term problem.

If the hormone method is used and the woman plans to use the pill in future, she should be sure that the next bleeding is truly a period before taking the first tablet. But if she takes it by the third day she can rely on the new method, as though she had used the first-day system described on page 44.

Above all, every woman having this treatment must be fully counselled and attend for follow-up to ensure it has worked . . .

How to obtain contraceptive advice
Already you may be thinking there seems a lot to take in about the pill. Actually, most advice about ordinary pill-taking can be summed up: continue taking your tablets according to the normal routine regardless of any development – except one of those mentioned on pages 61–2 – until you can talk to someone who knows the answers. All users of the pill should have access to such a trained person. This is usually a doctor but often a nurse, who can go over the points that apply to you personally.

What happens at the first family planning visit?

The exact procedure will depend quite a lot on where you go to get the pill. The arrangements vary: between different family doctors' surgeries, between different clinics, and in different countries. *As a minimum* you should always be asked some questions about your medical history in order to establish that you are suitable for the pill. Your age and smoking habits should be noted and you should be weighed and have your blood pressure checked.

In Britain and many other countries the addresses of family planning clinics are to be found in the telephone directory. If you go to one of them, you do not need to bring any doctor's letter with you. Your name is taken first at the reception desk – no objection whatsoever being made if you are unmarried – and your date of birth, address, and similar items are noted. A more confidential set of details is taken by a nurse in a separate side-room. She usually has a standard card to complete and all you have to do is answer her questions. She needs to know if you have had an abortion or miscarriage or ever had treatment for a sexually transmitted disease. The nurse plays a most important role in the modern family planning clinic. It is she who usually checks your weight and blood pressure, and tests your urine if necessary. (Specially trained nurses often do much more, including examinations.)

Then you will be called to see the doctor, everything again being completely confidential. There will normally be no problem about your partner coming in with you, if you would both like that. The doctor describes and discusses the various methods of family planning, and answers your questions about the pill if that is the method you are planning to use. Usually this can be done quite quickly. However, if there are any special points – for instance, if you are over 35, or are uneasy and feel ill-informed, or are under or not long past the legal age of consent – then time should be made for a longer discussion on all the pros and cons.

The examination

Contrary to what is believed by many women and by some doctors this is *not* a vital part of the first visit to start on the pill – apart, that is, from taking the blood pressure (which is indeed something you should insist on having done, see page 86). However, it is good preventive medicine to have the breasts examined to be sure there are no lumps, and to learn how to do this regularly yourself; to have a vaginal examination to check that the uterus, uterine tubes, and ovaries are normal; and to have a cervical smear test done. The latter should be done regularly in all sexually active women, especially pill-takers, but if you have not yet started having intercourse, there is absolutely no need for it at this stage.

If you have never had an internal examination, a brief description may be helpful. Women who were afraid of this beforehand usually wonder afterwards what they were worrying about. If you are relaxed it is entirely painless and very quick. In the *bimanual examination* the doctor uses both hands, the left hand on the abdomen and two gloved fingers of the right hand inside the vagina. The second part of the examination is with an instrument called a *speculum*. This takes up no more space in the vagina than the doctor's gloved two fingers did. It is designed to open out a little so that the walls of the vagina and the entrance to the uterus (the cervix) can be inspected. Using a flat wooden or plastic spatula the doctor may painlessly wipe some loose cells from the cervix on to a glass slide. After being fixed with a special solution this is sent to the laboratory to check that the cells are normal. This is all there is to the well-known *cervical smear* or '*Pap smear*' test. See also pages 21, 122, and 231, Questions 13 and 14.

The speculum is also used if swabs need to be taken and sent to the lab. This could be because you have noticed a big increase in the amount of normal vaginal discharge. With or without this, swabs are often taken if you have complained of soreness or itching or pain on intercourse.

Usually only three months' supply of the chosen pill are given at first. This is to make sure that you return for a further check-up, particularly of your blood pressure and weight, and for further supplies at that time. If you need special medical supervision for any reason, you may be asked to come back sooner.

Under-age sex

If you are under a certain age (16 in Britain), in many countries your partner will be breaking the law if you have intercourse. Plenty of couples do break this law. But that is not the only point – you may like to read again pages 21–3 and ask yourself the question there very carefully, about whether someone, perhaps you, might get hurt. You *could* be different, but the statistics do show that people who start having sex at this age are very likely to get hurt emotionally, and many of them end up in a marriage which they later regret. Then there are all the dangers of what used to be called VD (STDs, pages 19–21), which is so

67

common as to be difficult to avoid these days. It is also worth checking with yourself that you are not being *pressured* by boyfriends, girlfriends, or anyone at all. Although your friends, and some magazine articles, films, and TV programmes, seem to imply that 'everyone else does it', you are not a bit abnormal if you wait awhile. So if you are still thinking things over, you might – even if you are over the legal age, in fact – decide to do just that. If you are able to say 'no' you will save yourself from a lot of worry, and some risks.

On the other hand, if you are already having intercourse under age, know the dangers involved but feel that you will continue, I think you will find that most family planning doctors are prepared to prescribe you the pill – without moralizing. They will strongly encourage you to tell one or both of your parents, if you have not already done so. They might offer to do this for you if you would prefer: but only with your permission. If you think about it, it is really better all round to be open with your parents, and you could be agreeably surprised by their reaction.

But family planning doctors may sometimes think it better for you to take the pill even without the definite consent of your mother or father, if in their medical judgement you are seriously at risk of the even greater problem of an unwanted pregnancy.

I fully understand the complex problems there are here for both teenagers and their parents – writing now as a parent with a daughter who in due course will reach this age. Rather than say more here, and much more might be said, I would refer the interested reader to my postscript on page 247.

German measles (Rubella)

This illness, although it is so mild in the mother, can very seriously damage a developing baby during pregnancy. If you plan to have a baby at any time, it is sensible forward planning while you are safely protected against pregnancy to have the simple blood test to show whether you have immunity to Rubella. About one out of every four women in Britain who has this test done is found to be at risk. Do not rely on a history of German measles in the past: this is often wrong as other infections can imitate it. If you are not immune the vaccination is not painful and it is well worth having. Like the blood test it can easily be arranged by whoever supplies you with the pill. A most important point is that the vaccination itself could possibly also harm the baby if you fell pregnant during the next *three months*. Hence the logic of getting this matter sorted out while you are still on the pill or using another effective method.

To conclude, let me stress that family planning clinics are not concerned with whether you are married or single: they simply want to help you if you are at risk of an unwanted pregnancy. They are also very ready to help those who are a bit late, and think they might already be pregnant. It is never too late to go to a clinic and talk things through. If the early morning specimen of urine (which you should take with you in a clean glass bottle) shows that you are in fact pregnant, clinics can arrange appropriate counselling about the pregnancy. Most family planning nurses and doctors are easy to talk to, and are very helpful too if you have emotional problems or difficulties with any aspect of sex including intercourse itself. Special counselling can be arranged for couples where sex has become a problem.

Most of what I have described in the last few pages applies also if you go to your family doctor rather than to a clinic for your pills. The visits may tend to be briefer partly because he or she probably knows most of the important medical facts about you already. It is entirely up to you whether you prefer to go to a clinic or, like most women, to your doctor's office or surgery.

Follow-up visits

For pill-users the first return visit is commonly after three months, and then blood pressure and weight checks should be done as a routine every 6–12 months. An internal examination will only need to be done when you have the next regular cervical smear.

Last but not least

Never hesitate to go back to whoever prescribed your pills, immediately perhaps, or certainly sooner than your next routine visit, if you ever have doubts or anxieties about using the pill, or about any effect it seems to be having on you.

4

The pill: will it make me ill? Diseases of the circulation

The pregnancy-preventing or contraceptive effects of the pill were described in Chapter 2. The next two chapters summarize what we know about its other effects, starting here with changes in the chemistry of the body, and the very important effects the pill can have on the blood, heart, arteries, and veins.

We all know that reading any medical book tends to be rather alarming because we immediately begin to feel that we are suffering from most of the diseases it describes. Do you tend to expect the worst all the time? If so, remind yourself how many millions of women take the pill (page 3) and the majority stay entirely well. The list of side-effects which have ever been linked with the pill is a long one, and the next two chapters are bound to seem a bit threatening to some people. So be sure not to stop there but carry on and read Chapter 6, to help you to see things in proportion. The whole idea of this book is to 'spill the beans', to be as comprehensive as can be without turning into an encyclopaedia. But provided you are not someone who should avoid the method altogether for medical reasons – this is discussed in Chapter 7 – the chances of your getting any one of all the complications described here is very small.

Toxicity (poisoning)

One of the very good points about the pill is that unlike so many drugs on the market, and that includes many such as aspirin and paracetamol which can actually be bought over the counter, it seems to be almost impossible to take a fatal or even dangerous overdose. Let us be clear what this means: it is certainly possible for particular individuals unexpectedly to be very seriously harmed even by the normal doses of the pill. What I am saying here is that the general 'average person' – whether woman or man, or even a young child – is unlikely to be harmed even by taking a large handful of pills. Toddlers have been known to swallow dozens of their mothers' pills and apart from feeling or being rather sick at the time have ended up none the worse for the experience.

If the patient should be a baby girl, after a few days she may well have a 'period'. This is because the hormones have stimulated the lining of her tiny uterus. It therefore grows just as it would do 15 years later in the menstrual cycle, or if she took the pill. Hence, as her body gets rid of the swallowed pill hormones, a harmless hormone withdrawal bleed follows in the usual way. See pages 38–40.

Without emergency treatment, on the other hand, swallowing a similar number of iron or paracetamol (Panodol) tablets might be fatal. But obviously the pill, like all medicines, should be kept secure and out of the reach of children.

* Body chemistry

All the effects to be described later must have their ultimate explanation in the chemistry of the body. So it seems logical to make this our starting-point. More than 100 different laboratory tests on blood, urine, and other body fluids have given abnormal results in women on the pill. See Table 3 which shows just a few of the more important changes which have been described.

Many of the alterations are similar to those that would be found in normal pregnancy. This is not surprising. It was explained in Chapter 2 that, from the body's point of view, being on the pill in many ways mimics being pregnant. The fact that these changes are similar to those in pregnancy is somewhat reassuring. Pregnancy after all is a perfectly 'normal' condition and many women have a whole succession of pregnancies and live long and healthy lives. On the other hand, pregnancy is linked with an increased risk of several conditions including thrombosis which I shall be considering shortly in connection with the pill.

In spite of much research, we have as yet no idea what some of the changes in body chemistry mean in practice. Quite a number,

71

* **Table 3** Some changes in body chemistry

	Blood level	Remarks
Liver		
Liver functioning • *generally*	Altered in all users	These many changes cause no apparent harm to the liver itself, except in a tiny minority who develop jaundice. The liver is *involved*, however, in the production of most of the changes in blood level of substances shown in this table, including the important changes in blood sugar, fats, and clotting factors.
Albumin (*the main protein of blood*)	→↓→	
Transaminases (*special liver enzymes*)	Altered	
Amino acids ('building blocks' for body proteins) esp. Homocysteine	↓	
Blood sugar (glucose) after a meal	Altered (mostly ↑)	
Blood fats (lipids)	mostly ↑	These changes, hardly shown with the latest pills, may partly explain the increased risk of thrombosis in arteries. See page 75.
Clotting factors • *generally*		
Anti-thrombin III (special anti-clotting factor)	↓	See pages 77–8. Both the pill and smoking affect these interrelated systems, connected with the risk of thrombosis. Fibrinolysis is enhanced in the blood, but *reduced* in the vessel walls.
Fibrinolysis (the system to get rid of blood clots once formed)	↑	
Tendency for platelets to stick to each other (platelet aggregation)	↑	
Hormones		
Insulin	←→	
Growth hormone	←→	These hormone changes are thought to be connected with those affecting blood sugar and blood lipids (above).
Steroid hormones from adrenal gland	←→	
Thyroid gland hormones	←→	See page 75.
Luteinising hormone (LH)	←→	
Follicle stimulating hormone (FSH)	↓	Lowering the levels of these hormones is essential for the pill's contraceptive actions (see page 30).
Natural oestrogen	↓	
Natural progesterone	↓	
Prolactin	↑	Can cause milky fluid from breasts (see page 113).

Minerals and vitamins

Iron — This is a good effect (see page 76).

Copper, Zinc, Vitamins A, K, Riboflavine, folic acid, Vitamin B$_6$ (pyridoxine), Vitamin B$_{12}$ (cyanocobalamin), Vitamin C (ascorbic acid) — Effects unknown, but not believed to cause any health risk in most pill-users. Pyridoxine is discussed on page 93.

Binding globulins

These special substances carry hormones and minerals mostly in an inactive way in the blood. Because their levels increase in parallel with them, the *effective* blood levels of the hormones or minerals are not much altered.

Blood viscosity
Body water

This retention of fluids explains some of the weight gain blamed on the pill (see page 76). It means that women with certain heart and kidney diseases should avoid the pill.

Factors affecting blood pressure

Renin substrate	Altered
Renin activity	
Angiotensin II	
Output of the heart	

This is a very complicated story. Changes do not correlate as well as expected with the actual blood pressure levels (see page 86).

Immunity/allergy system

• Number of white blood cells	Altered
• Immunoglobulins (antibodies)	
• Function of the lymphocytes	See page 118.

73

Note: In the table arrow up ↑ means the level usually goes up, arrow down ↓ means the level tends to go down. 'Altered' means that the changes are known to be more complex, with both increases and decreases occurring in different substances within the system.

such as the changes in blood-clotting factors, have an obvious link with one of the known side-effects of the pill. Others which are so far unexplained may in due course be shown to lie behind a known or still unknown unwanted effect, or equally possibly some benefit of the pill. Others could turn out in the end to be entirely neutral changes.

As a general working rule, to play safe means that if we can measure any substance in the pill-user's body, we would like it to be normal – or as near normal as possible. So a lot of research is in progress to produce pills with minimal effects on the system. See pages 131–3, 162, 168, 191, 202–3.

One consequence of the changes in body chemistry is that whenever you visit a doctor it is most important to remind him of the fact if you are on the pill. This is particularly necessary if some specimen, such as a blood test, is going to be sent to a laboratory. The lab may be unable to interpret the results of the test satisfactorily unless this information is given.

* *Effects on the blood levels of sugar and of fats*

Many women on the pill show changes in their ability to deal with the rise in blood sugar that occurs after eating a meal. This is usually tested for by giving the patient a drink containing a measured amount of the most important blood sugar of the body (glucose) and then for up to three hours afterwards taking frequent blood and urine samples. This test is known as the oral Glucose Tolerance Test, and abnormal results like those in people with a very mild form of diabetes can be found in some pill-takers. Levels of the hormone insulin, which normally controls the level of blood glucose, tend to be higher than normal. See pages 81, 132. But none of the studies so far has shown that the fully developed condition of diabetes can be caused by the pill. Those few pill-users who do develop diabetes, and need injections of insulin or tablet treatment for it, are thought to be people who would in due course have been affected anyway.

Pill-users are also likely to have altered levels of certain fats (lipids) in the blood. This is sometimes called 'having a high blood cholesterol', but the changes are not simply increases: there are alterations in the proportions of the various different types of lipids. Similar changes have been found in some women
74

(and men) who have an above-average risk of heart attacks and strokes because of disease of their arteries. It is not known whether these changes mean the same when caused by the pill as when observed in studies of general populations. They happen to the majority of pill-takers without any apparent harmful effects. After stopping the pill they revert to normal within a few months. Similar changes in the lipids often occur in pregnancy.

There may be a particular small minority of women who are especially liable to unfavourable changes in their blood lipids. Not all can be identified in advance and there is much disagreement between the experts on this whole subject.

The experts do agree, however, that if even before taking the pill you are known to have one of the rare conditions of abnormal blood lipids – sometimes called hyperlipidaemia, or hypercholesterolaemia – then the combined pill should be avoided. See page 150.

* Effects on the body's own hormones

Some of the more important changes which have been discovered are listed in Table 3. See the various comments in the Remarks column.

* The thyroid gland

Although the total level of thyroid hormones rises in the blood, they are chiefly carried in an inactive way by the special thyroid hormone binding globulin (see Table 3). So their effects on the body are generally not altered. In fact there is now some reason to believe that the pill may actually protect the user against thyroid disease. This beneficial effect of the pill seems to apply to both over-activity and under-activity of the gland.

* Effects on blood levels of minerals and vitamins

The vitamin and mineral changes shown in Table 3 have not been shown to cause any harm at all to most women. They have caused concern to some nutritionists that pill-use might cause symptoms of deficiency diseases in poorly nourished women. However, studies among such women in developing countries have in general not confirmed this fear. And the World Health Organization found that women who were already short of vitamins showed no further decrease in measured levels after one year's use of the pill.

Folic acid and Vitamin B_{12} help to produce normal red blood cells. Anaemia due to the shortage of either of these substances has been described among pill-users, but very rarely and then only in women on poor diets. It might in fact have been a coincidence that they were pill-takers. The more frequent kind of anaemia due to shortage of iron is much *less* common. This is explained in the next chapter, by the fact that pill-users tend to have lighter periods and therefore to lose less iron from the body each month in the menstrual blood.

The lowered levels of most vitamins may even be necessary as the body adapts to being on the pill. *There may be no true shortage*. So pill-users need not take extra vitamins if they eat a normal diet, preferably including plenty of fruit and vegetables.

Taking too much extra vitamins might even do harm. For example, it is a quite common practice to take one gram a day of Vitamin C, in the belief that this will prevent or treat the common cold. *This is not recommended for pill-users*. The reason is that such high doses of Vitamin C very much increase the amount of ethinyloestradiol (page 34) absorbed in the digestive system. This is not good, as might be thought. It has the effect of turning a low-dose pill into a high-dose one, and results in more marked effects on the body chemistry – especially the clotting factors. This breaks that working rule on page 74.

Interestingly, intermittent use of a one-gram daily dose of Vitamin C has been found to cause breakthrough bleeding each time it is stopped. This is only to be expected, because it is like changing from a higher- to a lower-dose variety of pill, which commonly causes a small amount of bleeding, due to hormone withdrawal (see page 59).

If you are a strong believer in the value of Vitamin C, it would be best to take no more than a maximum of 300 mg per day.

For more about pyridoxine see page 93, and about folic acid see page 111.

Retention of fluid and weight gain

This occurs more in some women than others, and is due to some complicated adjustments to body chemistry among pill-users. Except in certain types of heart and kidney disease (in which

76

extra fluid can be dangerous and your doctor would not normally be recommending the pill) this seems to be quite harmless. It does, however, cause some of the weight gain for which the pill is often blamed, perhaps about one or two kilograms or so, just due to extra water being in the body. This is very temporary and the weight is lost if the pill is stopped. Some users notice that they shed the extra weight regularly during the 7-day break from pill-taking each month. Extra water is also kept in the body, for rather similar reasons, both towards the end of the normal menstrual cycle and in early pregnancy.

Weight gain after going on the pill can also result from an actual increase in body fat. This is largely due to an increase in appetite, particularly during the first three months. Watching your intake of calories is the only real answer to this: though this is easier said than done.

Gaining weight is one of the things which most puts women off the pill yet it is much less likely on the modern ultra-low-dose brands.

Disorders of the circulatory system: bloodstream, heart, arteries, and veins

Most of this next section has to do with one basic problem known as thrombosis, which is the formation of blood clots in arteries or veins. This causes most of the very rare major troubles blamed on the pill. But thrombosis is also more likely in pregnancy, which is of course avoided by taking the pill.

* *The ability to clot is a most important function of the blood*

Without it even a small injury to a blood-vessel could lead to the injured person bleeding to death. But the oestrogen of the pill tends to cause an increase in the blood levels of most of the important clotting factors and to reduce the amount of an important factor (anti-thrombin III) which tends to stop the clotting process. The pill also changes the functioning of the blood platelets. These are small particles which, among other things, have the ability to stick to each other at the start of clot formation. The tendency to platelet aggregation, as this process is called, is increased in heavy smokers. Recent laboratory research suggests it may also be increased by the combined pill, but probably by a different mechanism.

77

* These, among other changes, make clotting more likely to happen where it is *not* wanted, namely in uninjured arteries and veins. Yet if the changes occur to some extent in all pill-users, why do so few ever get any kind of thrombosis? An important reason for this seems to be that other systems are brought into play: particularly the one called fibrinolysis whereby any blood clots which appear in the circulation are removed as fast as they are formed. Thus often along with the increased tendency to clotting because of the raised clotting factors, there is at the same time a sufficient improvement of this process for getting rid of blood clots. Good health demands a balance between the two mechanisms. In pill-users it seems that this balance tends to be achieved by resetting them both at a higher level. Very interestingly, it has been found that this balancing increase in fibrinolysis tends not to happen in smokers, especially heavy smokers. If such women then take the pill, their increased clotting factors will no longer be counteracted by a better clot-removing system. This, along with the effect of smoking on platelets, may be part of the reason why smoking is such an important risk factor for thrombosis of the type occurring in arteries (see below).

Clotting can occur either in veins or arteries. Because these are everywhere in the body and the effect of a clot is to block the flow of blood at that point, what exactly happens will depend on whereabouts the blockage has occurred. If an *artery* is involved, then the part of the body supplied by that artery may lose its blood supply altogether and it can be severely damaged. *Veins* take the blood at low pressure back from different parts of the body to the heart. If they are blocked by a blood clot the local effects are usually less severe. The trouble with venous clots, however, is that they themselves may move through the bloodstream, by a process known as *embolism*, and finish up somewhere else, where they can do more harm. This is most commonly somewhere in the lungs.

Clotting in veins (venous thrombosis)

This was the first clotting problem to be linked with the pill and was recognized first in the large veins of the leg: the so-called deep veins. Given an increased level of clotting factors, the reason that clotting tends to occur in the legs is because the rate of flow tends to be slowest there. Lack of flow (stasis) is particularly likely if the pill-user is overweight, takes insufficient exercise, and above all if she is confined to bed by illness, operation, or accident.

As a rule, thrombosis of a deep vein shows up by pain and tenderness in the calf of the affected leg, aggravated if someone bends the ankle joint upwards. There may also be obvious swelling on that side. Whether or not there are these symptoms in the leg, rarely a piece of the blood clot may break off and after travelling in the great veins and right through the heart can finish up in the lung (*pulmonary embolism*). If the clot is big enough, this can – very rarely – even be fatal by stopping the blood flow through the lungs altogether. Otherwise there is a sharp pain in the chest, usually on one side or the other, worse at every breath, and sometimes a small amount of blood may be coughed up. The treatment, apart from stopping the pill *immediately, and for ever*, is usually by admission to hospital for treatment designed to 'thin' the blood. This is done by drugs called anti-coagulants, and sometimes by other treatments which can dissolve clots. Most exceptionally, in a severe case, an urgent operation on the chest to remove the clot may be required.

Like all the conditions in this chapter and the next, this chain of events can also happen in women who have never taken a pill in their lives, and in men. However, it is roughly four times more likely among women taking the pill than among non-users. It is connected with the oestrogen content – a fact which made earlier researchers exaggerate its dangers and take too little notice of the progestogen. We shall return to this point later (pages 131–3).

Apart from the pill itself, the factors which seem to make clotting in veins more likely are: obesity; confinement to bed; recent surgical operation (especially bone surgery); pregnancy; and past history of any form of thrombosis. Diabetes and high blood pressure are other factors associated with the risk. Thrombosis in veins is actually less common in people who have the blood group O. Fortunately, group O is in fact the commonest one, possessed by about half the population. Smoking is not connected with this kind of thrombosis, unlike the type discussed below, which can occur in arteries. The increased risk due to the pill is much reduced in modern low-oestrogen varieties: it is not related to duration of use, and it goes away quickly if the pill is stopped – certainly in about 4–6 weeks.

A note on varicose veins

Many women and some doctors wrongly think that you should always avoid the pill if you have varicose veins even if they have never caused any problems. This is just not so: the type of blood clotting I am describing here which can be dangerous starts in the *deep* veins, particularly of the calf.

Many women who would like to use the pill are frightened to take it because of really almost microscopic varicose veins. Some of them then actually finish up with the tragedy of an unwanted pregnancy. *Provided* the other risk factors which were listed above do not apply to you, and especially if you are not overweight, moderate varicose veins with no signs of any past thrombosis need not stop you going on the pill. You may notice that they become a little more prominent and that you perhaps get some aching in legs, particularly if you have to stand a long time. However, should you, without any obvious explanation for it (such as an injection or pressure from a plaster cast), suffer from 'phlebitis' in a vein, which involves thrombosis, you should stop the pill. You also should never take it again in case you were to have a clot somewhere more important next time.

Injection treatment for varicose veins works by causing clotting in them, after which the body causes scarring to seal them up. To prevent this being overdone, you should stop the pill a month beforehand, stay off it during the period that you visit your doctor's surgery or the out-patient department for the treatment, and ideally for three months afterwards. During all this time you will of course need to use some other reliable method of family planning. As the clotting was caused deliberately, this treatment should not stop you going on the pill once again, provided your doctor agrees.

Clotting in arteries (arterial thrombosis)

The main reason why clotting in arteries occurs is because of a disease of the walls of the arteries which is often called arteriosclerosis ('hardening of the arteries') or more properly atherosclerosis. This disease affects almost everyone in due course, men usually at a younger age than women. In the more developed countries of the world it has usually started by the age of 20, and gets more marked as the individual gets older, especially if he or she is a smoker. It affects some much more than others, and one important factor seems to be high levels or an abnormal ratio of the levels of the various blood lipids mentioned earlier. The tendency to high blood sugar and insulin levels in some pill-takers (page 74) may be relevant too, because similar changes are found in the blood of diabetics, who are particularly prone to atherosclerosis.

The changes in blood-clotting factors, especially those which affect the blood platelets, are also important. Given the fact that the walls of an artery have been damaged by atherosclerosis, clotting on the surface of the roughened bit of the wall can then occur and eventually this may block up the artery altogether. If it is an important one, such as an artery supplying the heart, the results can be very serious – i.e. a coronary thrombosis or heart attack. If the artery supplies part of the brain, then a cerebral thrombosis may result with the production of one type of stroke. Once again it is important to realize that any of these events can happen, unfortunately, to women who have never taken a single pill in their lives and to *men*. What the pill seems to do is to increase the chance of arterial blood clotting above the normal odds. But in most women under the age of 35, especially if they do not smoke, the increased risk is very small.

Coronary thrombosis (heart attack)

The pill is only one of many factors which make heart attacks more likely, and indeed a less important one than some of those in the list which follows.

Risk factors for arterial thrombosis:

1. *Abnormal blood fats.* As discussed earlier, there is a group of people who have a 'high blood cholesterol' from birth and should never take the pill. Many of them know about this, but a lot more do not: the appropriate blood tests need to be done if a near-relative (especially mother, father, sister, or brother) suffered a first heart attack or other arterial thrombosis under the age of 45. (See also pages 74 and 132.)

2. *Diabetes requiring treatment.*

3. *High blood pressure, bad enough for treatment.* A past history of blood pressure problems in pregnancy – properly called pre-eclamptic toxaemia – may also be a factor, though this is debatable. It is probably only important when it happens to someone who already had a blood pressure problem even when not pregnant (though she may not have known about it then). So the pill need not be avoided if you have a history of blood pressure in pregnancy. It will just be important to keep a closer eye than usual on your blood pressure especially in the early months of pill-taking.

4. *Cigarette-smoking,* especially if heavy. In one study which included 64 women under 40 who suffered heart attacks, 60 were smokers. Only 17 were pill-users, all of them smokers. Thus there were no cases in pill-users unless they *also* smoked.

5. *Increasing age,* especially beyond 35 to 40.

These are the main factors about which there is general agreement that they increase the risk of heart attacks.

6. *Obesity* is also a factor increasing the risk, but it possibly does not act independently. In other words, many experts believe that it tends to go along with or have a hand in causing some of the other factors mentioned such as abnormal blood fats, or diabetes, and these explain the extra risk.

7. Another factor is the possession of a *blood group other than group O*. (The other groups in this system are groups A, B, and AB.) In other words, blood group O seems to give a bit of protection against clotting in arteries as well as veins. Though not routinely tested for, the presence of group O can help tip the balance about using the pill in a borderline case – e.g. a woman with one or more of risk factors 1–6.

The important thing to understand about these factors is that if more than one applies to a particular woman there is a dramatic increase in the risk she runs. Let us take as an example a healthy 25-year-old woman who is not a diabetic, has normal blood fat levels and blood pressure, and does not smoke. If she goes on a combined pill the minute risk of a heart attack which she ran before is, in round figures, about doubled. If instead she starts to smoke cigarettes her chances of a coronary are something like three times greater than before, depending on how many she smokes. But if she swallows a daily pill and also smokes more than 15 cigarettes a day her risk goes up by two for the pill *multiplied* by three (for the smoking), to six times the initial value. Double that if her daily consumption is 30 cigarettes. What would happen if she had a third risk factor, say a sufficiently raised blood pressure to add a further five-times risk? Multiplying again, she would then be five times twelve or 60 times less safe than a healthy non-smoker with normal blood pressure not taking the pill. Yet, as we saw, just taking the pill only about doubled her risk.

All these figures are very, very approximate. Research so far cannot give precise estimates of the risks, and they are only averages anyway whereas every pill-user is a unique individual.

The risk factors in the list above are also relevant (some more than others) to the causation of other forms of thrombosis in arteries – see below. If you look again at the list it will be clear that there is not a lot you can do about several of them. If you have that high blood cholesterol condition which runs in families, or you are unlucky enough to have diabetes, or have now developed high blood pressure – apart from taking your doctor's advice and treatment, relaxing a bit, and perhaps taking more exercise, there is not much you can do about the situation. Nor, more's the pity, can you make yourself younger or change your blood group! If you are overweight you ought to be able to return to the ideal weight for your height by dieting, and this is well worth doing anyway. But the number one risk factor that you can in theory do something about, and which is perhaps the most common and may well be one of the most important, is of course *smoking*. As one researcher has said, summarizing a lot of research by experts in many different countries, coronary thrombosis 'in otherwise healthy pre-menopausal women is almost exclusively an illness of cigarette smokers'.

Clotting in the arteries of the brain (cerebral thrombosis)

This can cause one type of *stroke:* very suddenly the person notices weakness or marked tingling, leading to loss of all sensation or the ability to move the muscles on one side of the body; or loss of the power of normal speech; with perhaps a headache on the opposite side of the head to the side of the body affected. Other symptoms may be produced, depending on which part of the brain is damaged. Sometimes there can be almost complete recovery, but sadly some people are left with permanent loss of power or feeling on one side and perhaps impairment of their speech. Stroke in general is very rare among women under the age of 40. However, we now know that the pill increases the risk, both of this type of stroke and of the type due to bleeding into the brain which can often be very difficult to distinguish from it (described below). Interestingly, although the thrombosis occurs in arteries, no connection between this type of stroke and smoking has yet been shown – but see below.

Strokes caused by bleeding

Two varieties of strokes due to bleeding appear to be more likely among pill-users. One is *intracerebral haemorrhage* (bleeding into the substance of the brain) causing damage and similar symptoms to those after thrombosis in the arteries supplying the same part of the brain. The other is known as *subarachnoid haemorrhage*, or bleeding into the cerebro-spinal fluid which surrounds the brain and spinal cord. This type leads to rapid and often prolonged loss of consciousness, from which the patient may or may not make a slow and not always complete recovery following medical or surgical treatment. Both these rare catastrophes are due to a localized weakness of the wall of an artery in the brain giving way. There seems to be a very clear link between these types of stroke and smoking. In one study, eight of nine current or past users of the pill who had a subarachnoid haemorrhage were also smokers. High blood pressure, whether or not the pill has ever been used, is even more important. Some people are born with a weakness somewhere in a brain artery: raised pressure in that artery will make it more likely to give way. A British study, published in December 1979, concluded from all the known facts that subarachnoid haemorrhage 'should thus probably not be regarded as a serious cause for concern in healthy women using the pill, provided their blood pressure remains in the normal range' (see pages 86–7).

Prevention of strokes

Sometimes a stroke may be avoidable by prompt action, mainly by stopping the pill if ever the blood pressure is found to be too high (pages 87, 150) and also if certain unusual symptoms appear. A few migraine sufferers notice while taking the pill a marked change in the pattern of their migraine, so that it becomes more *focal* as it is called, with clear-cut localization of their symptoms to one part or function of the body. With or sometimes without a migraine headache, such symptoms have been noticed in the past, in some women, some hours or a few days before an actual stroke occurred. They include: *sudden* onset of short-lived but marked tingling and weakness affecting one side of the body or one limb only; brief loss of one half of the field of vision; a fleeting difficulty in speaking normally; a first-ever shaking attack like an epileptic fit; or loss of consciousness.

NB *Headache on one side of the head is not on the list, as this is normal in migraine.*

Such symptoms just might mean that there is a temporary loss of blood supply to part of the brain. With or without a headache they should be treated as an early warning and the pill stopped at once, probably for ever. This may prevent blockage to an artery from becoming permanent.

However, strokes are very uncommon, so there could well be a quite different explanation in your case. When in doubt, discuss any strange symptoms promptly with your doctor (see page 61).

* Thrombosis in other parts of the body

As there are arteries and veins everywhere, so thrombosis can affect other organs than those mentioned so far.

* *Mesenteric thrombosis* is the name given to clotting in an artery or vein which supplies the bowel.

- If a large *artery* is affected an emergency operation may be required to remove the dead bowel and stitch together the live parts each side of it. If the bowel survives, an unusual condition called ischaemic colitis can occur instead, causing longer-term pain and bloody diarrhoea. This very rare problem responds to stopping the pill.
- If one of the main *veins* leading from the bowel is affected, the results can vary between nothing, because the other veins take over, and serious, because of interference with the flow of blood taking absorbed food substances to the liver. There have also been isolated reports of blockage in the veins the other side of the liver, on the way back to the heart.

* *The eyes.* Rarely, venous or arterial thrombosis (*or* bleeding) can cause damage to a part or all of the retina (the light-sensitive part at the back of the eye). This causes loss of vision in the affected eye, which is a disaster if it should be permanent: but it may be only temporary if the pill is stopped and expert treatment started at once.

Raised blood pressure

In most pill-users there is a measurable slight rise in blood pressure. However, in only one or two women out of every forty who take the pill does this reach the level at which doctors term it hypertension. The reason why the rest are not more affected is still not clear. There are certainly changes in the circulation and in body chemistry (see Table 3) which may be involved, but those which have been measured often happen also in pill-users without a particularly high blood pressure. Some individuals are known to be more prone generally to raised blood pressure: those with a history of it in their family, those who have had kidney disease, and some black people. The pill may 'bring out' the blood pressure problem in such women, particularly as they get older. One group of researchers has also shown that women with hypertension on the pill have higher levels of the hormone ethinyloestradiol in their blood than other pill-users. So perhaps the few individuals who develop this problem are exceptional in the way their bodies absorb and handle the pill's hormones.

Whatever the reason, there are two main points about raised blood pressure. First, it usually does *not* make you feel at all unwell. Second, when large groups of both men and women with even very mild hypertension have been followed up, they have not remained as healthy over the years as comparison groups with entirely normal blood pressure readings. Blood pressure seems to be linked with nearly all the diseases of the circulatory system and is often a feature of people who later suffer thrombosis in veins, heart attacks, and strokes. It also has the risk itself of becoming uncontrollable, even with drugs, leading to malignant hypertension which is very rare but fatal.

As raised blood pressure is something that can be readily detected, it can be used as an early warning sign of other circulation problems with which it seems to be linked. It is obviously vital, therefore, if you use the pill that you have your blood pressure taken regularly. The pressure is measured in the main artery of the arm, the brachial artery. The highest (systolic) pressure reached in that artery during each pumping action of the heart is the first figure that doctors quote, and should not normally be above about 140 mm of mercury. The lowest pressure reached before the next heartbeat is the other measurement, the diastolic pressure, and should not be above 90 mm. Several readings above these levels are necessary before mild hypertension is diagnosed. Careful medical supervision is then required, and if there are any other risk factors the pill should be discontinued. The pill usually has to be stopped anyway if the upper figure reaches 160 mm or the lower 95 mm or more (these figures are those used by the World Health Organization to define clinical hypertension). Just stopping the pill generally brings the blood pressure back to normal within a month or two. Further treatment (with drugs) is rarely required for women during the child-bearing years. All brands of the combined pill tend to cause a recurrence of the problem, but the progestogen-only pill (Chapter 8) may be tried.

The Study of the British Royal College of General Practitioners

Much of the information for this chapter and the next comes from the Oral Contraception Study organized by the Royal College of General Practitioners (RCGP). The Study began in 1968 when about 23,000 pill-users from the practices of 1,400 family doctors all over Britain were matched up with another 23,000 similar women who were not taking the pill. Ever since that time every episode of disease, treated at home or requiring hospital admission, and all pregnancies and of course deaths were recorded. Many women discontinued the pill for one reason or another, so that eventually there were three groups: pill-takers, ex-takers, and never-users. The ex-takers have been studied carefully for any possible harmful effects of the pill which might carry on even after it was stopped.

Two similar studies also began in 1968. One, referred to as the Oxford/FPA Study, was organized by the British Family Planning Association working with Professor Vessey of Oxford University. Full details were obtained of all the hospital attendances of 17,032 women who were recruited between 1968 and 1974 from FPA clinics throughout Britain. A little over half the women were on the pill when first seen, the others used the cap or an intra-uterine device (IUD).

The Walnut Creek Study is named after a suburban township near San Francisco, California. Between 1968 and 1972, 16,638 women had a general health check-up provided by the Kaiser-Permanente Medical Care Program at Walnut Creek. They were subsequently followed up until 1977 and their health details were analysed. Those who had used or were currently using the pill were compared with the remainder, whose methods of con-traception (if any) were not recorded. (This is a weakness of the Walnut Creek Study and applies to the RCGP one as well.)

The findings of these three groups of researchers differ in some details but agree in most important respects. As the RCGP group studied the largest number, its results more commonly have statistical significance. But most weight is given in this book, as it should be, to those findings which are confirmed by other studies (such as the other two mentioned), as well as other types of research in different populations.

The RCGP researchers concluded that the overall death rate due to diseases of the circulation was about four times greater in 'ever-users' (55) of the pill than 'never-users' (10). The numbers in brackets are the actual numbers of deaths, totalling 65. That is not a large number out of the 46,377 studied, for an average of just under seven years (322,438 woman-years of observation). Among the individual circulatory conditions mentioned earlier in this chapter, some increase more than fourfold, some less, than the overall fourfold increase. But the diseases are fortu-nately all so rare in young women that these increased rates are not as bad as they sound at first. Please see page 141 for discussion of this important subject of *attributable risk*.

Among current users the RCGP researchers could find no effect of duration of use on the risk of circulatory disease. This is a good piece of news which emerged only in their latest report (1981). At the age of 30 a woman's risk is the same whether she has previously taken the pill for one year or for ten years. Although the last statement is believed to be true for her risk as long as she stays on the pill, there may be an effect of duration of use on the (smaller) ex-use risks discussed on page 128.

The two most important causes of death in the RCGP Study

88

were both arterial diseases: coronary thrombosis (page 81) and subarachnoid haemorrhage (page 84). Both are also linked with smoking. Other researchers agree about the first, but tend to find a lower risk of the second disease (about 1.5 times increase in risk for pill-users rather than the four times greater rate suggested by the RCGP).

The overall death rates hide within them very different risks for different sub-groups of pill-users (see page 141). As the main serious problem is arterial disease, the women chiefly at risk are those with any of the risk factors listed on pages 81–2.

Smoking, age, and the pill – THE PILL MAKES YOUR SMOKING EVEN MORE DANGEROUS

All studies agree that the pill's hazards are heavily concentrated in cigarette smokers and older women. No less than 54 of the total 65 deaths in the RCGP Study (83 per cent) were in women over 35. Only two of the 55 deaths in pill-users were in women who were neither over 35 nor smokers, and two-thirds of them were both. Smoking seems to do two things: not only does it increase the risk of getting an arterial disease, it also makes the attack more likely to be fatal.

The Walnut Creek researchers were even more emphatic. They could show the risk for pill-users who were also smokers, and for non-pill-users who smoked. In the absence of smoking, however, it seemed that the pill was not linked to circulatory disease at all. Actually this study does *not* prove complete absence of risk because all the numbers were too small to be statistically valid. But it certainly adds up to good news for young women who do not smoke cigarettes.

Table 4 is one of the most important in this book, so please study it carefully. It sets out the risks of taking the pill according to your age and whether you are a non-smoker, a light smoker (0–14 cigarettes per day), or a heavy smoker (15 or more per day). The fewer the stars, the lower the risk.

One of the first things to notice from Table 4 is that *heavy smoking effectively makes you 5–10 years older than you really are.* For example, a heavy smoker under 30 is already taking as big a risk by going on the pill as if she were a non-smoker of age

89

Table 4 Smoking habits and age. Risk of disease of the circulation if also using the ordinary combined pill

Age	Below 30	30–34	35–39	40–44	45+
Heavy smoker: 15 per day or more	**	***	****	*****	*****
Smoker: under 15 per day	*	**	***(*)	*****	*****
Non-smoker, without other predisposing risk factors (see page 81)	*	*	**	***(*)	*****

* Low risk
** Moderate risk
*** Fairly high risk – *may* be acceptable
**** High risk – rarely acceptable
***** Too high risk! (unacceptable except very rarely for supervised hormone *treatment*)

Note: Stars have been used because the exact figures for these categories are not all available. As a rough guide, one star (*) means that the annual 'betting odds' on survival are between 100,000 to 1 and 50,000 to 1. Five stars (*****) means the odds are 100 times worse – between 1,000 to 1 and 500 to 1. So the pill should not normally be prescribed to women in the four- and five-star categories.

35 to 39 (2 stars). At 31 she has reached the 3-star level of risk that means she should consider very seriously whether she should even continue using the pill. This is a dilemma that does not have to be faced by a non-smoker until she is around 40.

Figure 13 shows this graphically. Whatever level of risk a pill-user is prepared to accept, if she is a smoker she will reach it 5–10 years sooner. In the example shown, an overall annual risk of 20 per 100,000 women (i.e. betting odds on survival 5,000 to 1) is reached at about age 32, rather than 39 for a non-smoker.

It may well be that some heavy smokers will react by saying 'Obviously I shall have to avoid the pill.' To continue puffing away, in the face of the known facts about the relative dangers of the pill and of smoking, is to 'strain out a mosquito and swallow a camel'; or a bit like a stunt motor-cyclist refusing to play golf in case she might get hurt!

Smoking in effect ages your arteries and increases the risk of most diseases of the circulation for all women (and men), regardless of their method of family planning. If you carry on smoking, you are continuing with at least a pill's-worth of risk of heart disease and strokes – more than a pill's-worth in fact if you smoke heavily. On top of that you are accepting some pretty

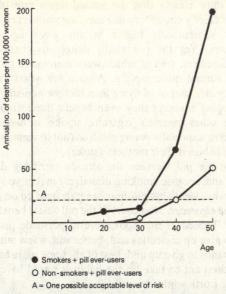

Fig. 13 Influence of pill-use, smoking, and age, on overall death rates due to diseases of the circulation. Based on figures from the RCGP report (1981).

frightening hazards, including bronchitis, gangrene of the legs, and cancer of the lung, larynx, bladder, and cervix. (The last two, and others not listed, are by the effect of chemicals absorbed from the smoke into the bloodstream, see page 41.) About 25 per cent of smokers die earlier than they otherwise would of a disease related to smoking.

Of course, you can get injured by a golf ball, and the pill certainly does have problems. But if you add up all the problems mentioned in this chapter and the next, it still does not put the pill into the same league as the cigarette. And the trouble is that if you add the pill to your cigarettes, you make smoking even more dangerous than it would otherwise be.

The obvious if difficult answer is to get rid of the smoking – and if you look again at Table 4, you can see at once that you can shed up to 2 stars of pill-taking risk in each age-group from 30 to 44 by becoming a non-smoker. *It is always worth giving up.*

91

Statistics show clearly that the annual death rate (due to *all* causes but chiefly circulatory diseases) for smokers of either sex is always substantially higher at any given age than for non-smokers. Yet the potentially dangerous changes in the blood of smokers, two of which were mentioned on page 78, revert to normal quite rapidly. After a few years ex-smokers have no greater chance of dying than lifetime non-smokers.

By stopping smoking they even benefit those around them. Breathing other people's cigarette smoke is dangerous for non-smokers, especially young children (not to mention the risks to *unborn* babies if their mothers smoke).

Because the pill worsens the already terrifying dangers of smoking, and because smoking effectively makes you ten years older anyway, *ideally no pill-user, whether aged 20 or 35, should ever smoke cigarettes*. Non-users of the pill would benefit as well, of course. Indeed, if this book were to persuade just a dozen women to give up cigarettes and, better still, a few more to help their husbands to give up and, best of all, some more to persuade their children not to take up the habit, it would have achieved something worth while.

5

Other effects of the pill

This chapter is like a conducted tour of the systems of the body, starting at the head and more or less working downwards. At the end there are some miscellaneous subjects which do not readily fit in elsewhere. Conditions which were dealt with in the last chapter because they were primarily caused by a disorder of the circulation are only cross-referenced. This applies, for example, to strokes, which are disorders of the brain and central nervous system but are caused by arterial disease and have therefore already been discussed.

Within each system, the more common known unwanted effects are considered before those that are rare, followed by the known good effects.

The brain and central nervous system

Depression

This is a most complicated subject. Firstly, depression which comes on regularly pre-menstrually in the normal menstrual cycle is, naturally, most commonly improved by the pill. Secondly, there is no suggestion from any of the research that the pill increases the risk of depression, or of any type of mental disorder, which is so severe as to require a specialist opinion or admission to hospital. However, most researchers do find that a few more than the expected number of women using the pill complain of mild or moderate depression. And there could sometimes be an explanation in body chemistry because, as shown in Table 3, pyridoxine (Vitamin B_6) levels are lowered in the blood of some depressed pill-users. This vitamin is known to be involved in producing certain amines of the brain, substances which affect how it functions. Depressed pill-users with lowered levels of pyridoxine, but not those who were equally depressed with normal blood levels of the vitamin, did notice an improvement in one study in which they were given extra amounts of this vitamin every day. But the experts are very divided as to whether it is a good idea to make it a routine that pill-users who complain of depression are given pyridoxine. The treatment would not benefit those who did not lack this vitamin. Those who lack it might be helped, and some doctors therefore prescribe it. A dose of 25 mg per day is plenty and should do no harm so far as we know. Foods that are rich in pyridoxine include wheatgerm, liver, meats, fish, milk, bananas and peanuts.

As a matter of fact, there are reasons for questioning how much of the increase in depression reported among pill-users is really due to the pill. The excess rate in the RCGP Study was only about 30 per cent. Now depression is very common, and affects practically everyone – men as well as women – at some time or another. The pill is commonly used, so depression and use of the pill might well come together by coincidence. The pill may be blamed when really the depression is due to a combination of factors in the woman's whole life. But these may be so hard to tackle that it is very understandable to hope that stopping the pill will be the answer.

Another point is that the pill-users in the RCGP Study had to go to their doctor more often than the non-users just to pick up their prescriptions, and so would be more likely to mention the fact if they were depressed. This could lead to a bias against the pill. If for the sake of argument we blame the pill for the whole 30 per cent excess noted among users, that still means that out of every 130 depressed pill-users 100 cannot really blame their depression on the method.

The pill has such a reputation for causing depression that this is the commonest reason given by women who stop using it. Many could be giving it up unnecessarily. (Some of them may end up with a very depressing unplanned pregnancy.) Having said that, it is still true that there is a group of women who do find that their mood improves dramatically when they stop taking the pill and worsens whenever they start it again.

So, what should you do if you become depressed while taking

the pill? The best advice is to discuss the whole matter with your doctor. Moving to an ultra-low-dose pill may help, or to one containing a different progestogen, and this is certainly worth a try if this is the only problem before transferring to another method altogether. Your doctor might suggest treatment with pyridoxine, or perhaps with some anti-depressant or tranquillizer: if so, be sure to discuss whether the pill and the new medicine might interfere with each other's actions (see page 56). Finally, take heart from the fact that mild and moderate attacks of depression are not 'life sentences' and usually you can expect to feel better before too many months have gone by.

Loss of libido (interest in sex)

This can happen because of depression, but also for other reasons. Few people realize how common it is, especially after a recent pregnancy. Many women start taking the pill after having a baby, and blame the pill for the depression and loss of libido that follows when it is really part of the post-natal 'blues'.

Another possible explanation is that some women still feel that sex is primarily for babies, and as taking the pill makes pregnancy extremely unlikely, they lose their interest in love-making. However, these two explanations are not the whole story. Like depression, it is undeniable that some cases are indeed caused by the pill. One simple diagnosis can be that the vagina seems drier in some women due to some loss of the natural lubrication. If this is the problem it can be helped considerably by using something like a jelly lubricant regularly before intercourse. Actually, many women report an improvement in their sex lives once they go on the pill and most surveys have shown that, in general, pill-users have more intercourse each month. This may be because the pill avoids the 'turn-off' effect which some couples find with alternative methods. Or it may reduce the regular loss of libido due to pre-menstrual tension which many women get in their (so-called) normal menstrual cycles.

So once again, take heart if you do go through a phase of lost interest in sex on the pill. Discuss the whole matter with your doctor. Transferring to a more oestrogen-dominant pill may help (pages 178–9). In a few cases the doctor may recommend some special sessions of counselling for you and your partner, to improve your general and sexual relationship. Only rarely should it be necessary for you to give up the pill solely for this reason.

Migraine

Migraines are periodic, very variable, often severe, and usually one-sided headaches, linked with sickness or actual vomiting. There are commonly other symptoms like intolerance of bright lights or noise and short-lived disturbances of vision. There is much disagreement between doctors as to what causes migraines. In many women they are thought to be due to an alteration in the responsiveness of the blood-vessels of the brain to those special substances called amines (see page 93). The pill may cause migraines by affecting these amines, perhaps partly because of its effects on the vitamin pyridoxine. Another important factor can be amines coming in the diet: for instance, cheese, chocolate, sherry, and red wine are all rich in one of them (tyramine), and can all precipitate migraine in some women. Allergy may also be a factor in some people, smoking is important, and three out of every four migraine sufferers have a family history of some relative with the same problem.

A very few women on the pill actually report some improvement in their migraines. Rather more say that the pill makes their attacks more frequent, or has even brought this problem on for the very first time. One of the most common patterns is for the headaches to occur during the seven days while the woman is not taking tablets, probably because of the sudden drop in the hormone levels. A possible short-term solution is then to take an ultra-low-dose combined pill on the three-monthly basis described on page 42. For this purpose, a pill from near the bottom of one of the 'ladders' discussed in Chapter 7 (Figure 15, pages 165–7) should be chosen and even then this approach cannot be recommended for very long-term use because of the extra hormone-taking that it will obviously involve. Transferring to a progestogen-only pill (Chapter 8) can sometimes help as this is also taken every day with no pill-free weeks.

For all types of migraine, avoiding various foods, cigarettes, and stressful situations can help. It can be a miserable complaint. In practice, the majority of sufferers from true migraines give the pill up altogether. This is indeed recommended for those who develop migraines for the first time while taking the pill, or who require to take ergotamine-containing drugs during attacks (Table 2b, page 59). The pill should also be stopped immediately and you should discuss the matter promptly with a doctor if:

(a) pre-existing migraine worsens to produce a headache which simply gets worse and worse and worse as the hours go by, or

(b) you begin to get very *localized* or so-called 'focal' symptoms (but *not* just a one-sided headache).

Examples of the kind of symptoms and the reasons for acting promptly in this way are given on page 85.

Headaches

Ordinary (non-migraine) headaches are extremely common in women not taking the pill and also in men. Thus it is hard to know how much the pill can really be blamed for the headaches pill-users may get. After depression, this was the second commonest reason women gave for giving up the method in the RCGP Study. Apart from taking pain-killers if necessary, the treatment is to use the very lowest-dose pill that suits you in other ways. If they happen mostly during the pill-free week, your doctor may recommend the tricycle regime (page 42). You could change the progestogen (transferring to a different 'ladder' – see Figure 15); or possibly transfer to the progestogen-only pill. It would be rather unusual for you to have to give up the method for this reason alone.

* *Epilepsy*

There is no suggestion that the pill *causes* epilepsy. In fact many sufferers report fewer attacks when they go on the pill. However, a very few do get more frequent epileptic attacks, and may have to give up the pill. There is also the distinct possibility that the tablets they take to control fits may interfere with the hormones of the pill once absorbed into the body, and reduce the protection it provides against pregnancy (see page 56). There is one anti-epileptic drug (sodium valproate) which seems not to do this, but it is not the ideal drug for all patients. Those who are on the other treatments should discuss the whole matter with their doctor. They may decide to use another method such as the IUD, but the pill can still be some women's best choice of family planning method. If so it should definitely be one of the ones containing 50 micrograms of oestrogen from Table 9 (page 163). The woman should be more than usually careful to take her tablets regularly and will also have to report promptly back to the surgery or clinic should she develop 'breakthrough' bleeding or miss a period (see page 57).

See also pages 83–5 for *strokes*.

* Chorea

This rare condition causes the patient to make strange uncontrolled fidgety movements of the head, arms, and legs. It may have occurred in the past, during an attack of rheumatic fever or in pregnancy. With or without such a history, it has been found to happen in one or two pill-users. It always clears up if the pill is discontinued.

* Benign Intracranial Pressure (BICP)

Neurologists report that pill-use is common among those few young thin women who give a strange story that they notice headache and a blind spot in their field of vision on exercise. If they also have swelling of the optic nerves when the light-sensitive retina at the back of their eyes is examined (papilloedema), the condition is called BICP. It always gets better if the pill is stopped – as it should be following rule 8 on page 62.

The eyes

Problems with contact lenses

Some contact-lens-users find that their eyes get sore for the first time when they start the pill. A possible reason seems to be that there is a slight increase in the amount of fluid in the cornea (the transparent covering in front of the iris). If the eyes do become really uncomfortable, it is important that vanity does not make you persevere too long and you take the lenses out to give the eyes a rest. (It is possible otherwise to damage the surface of the sensitive cornea.) Then you should discuss the matter with your optician. Although this complaint is definitely less common with modern lenses, and with modern ultra-low-dose pills, a few women do have to make a straight choice: either the pill or their contact lenses.

* *Other eye problems*

A couple of reports suggest that long-term pill-users cannot see the colour blue as well as non-users. This was something that showed up on specialized testing, and not something of which the women themselves complained.

Quite a range of other eye problems have been reported in women who were taking the pill. In many of them pill-use may well have been coincidental. For example, no link has been proved between the pill and glaucoma (in which there is a rise in the pressure of the fluid within the eyeball).

See also page 86 for *retinal thrombosis/bleeding*.

The respiratory system: air passages and lungs

Allergic rhinitis (hay fever)

This can sometimes become a problem for the first time when a woman starts taking the pill. The pill seems to be able to alter the immune systems of the body (see Table 3 and page 118), so this could be a genuine effect of the pill, though not yet proved to be so.

Asthma

This does not appear to start for the first time more commonly in pill-users than other women, probably because it is a problem which tends to run in families and rarely starts for the first time in adults. Some women with asthma notice that their symptoms are improved on the pill, some that they are worsened. In the majority there is no change. So if the method suits in other ways it is well worth a try.

See also page 79 for *pulmonary embolism*.

Disorders of the digestive system

Nausea (queasiness)

With modern pills this is quite uncommon except in women who are underweight – including therefore many pill-users from the developing world. If it occurs, it is experienced particularly during the first few days of pill-taking, from each of the first two or three packets. Perseverance, or taking the pills at bedtime so

99

that you are asleep when the symptom appears, or moving down to the lowest-dose pill which otherwise suits you, should all be tried before giving up. Do not forget the possibility that the nausea might be due to pregnancy, of course, particularly if it appears for the first time after several months' use of the method. See your doctor if in any doubt.

Duodenal ulcers

Here we have a possible good effect of the pill. Both the RCGP Study and the Oxford/FPA Study are agreed that women on the pill were less likely than non-users to require treatment for severe indigestion due to this type of ulcer. However, it is hard to rule out the possibility that the anxious person who is prone to get such ulcers will also be particularly unlikely to use the pill.

Crohn's disease

This uncommon bowel disease causes pain and diarrhoea. It appears that one form of it occurs more frequently in pill-takers; but if the pill is stopped, complete recovery is the rule.

See page 85 for *mesenteric thrombosis*.

The liver and gall-bladder

The liver has many special *receptors* for sex hormones, and therefore its many functions are often influenced by the pill (see Table 3). The alterations, in clotting factors for example, mean that the liver is probably at the back of most of the unwanted effects of the pill which occur elsewhere. But in most women the liver itself is not apparently harmed in any way.

See page 124 for *liver tumours*.

Jaundice

This is the liver disease which makes the skin and eyeballs go a yellow colour. The reason for this is an increase in the amount of a yellow substance called bilirubin in the blood. Bilirubin is normally present in the bile, which is a fluid produced by the liver and carried in ducts to the small bowel. This fluid helps in the digestion of food. A very small number of pill-users may get jaundice of a special type, due to blockage within the substance of the liver to this flow of bile. There is then back-pressure so some of the bile spills over into the general bloodstream, so causing yellowness and also itching. The same type of jaundice can occur sometimes in late pregnancy. In fact, if you had this jaundice in pregnancy, or if you had troublesome itching in late pregnancy which often has the same explanation, then you will be advised to avoid using the combined pill altogether in case it causes a recurrence.

Gallstones

The gall-bladder is the reservoir for bile. Bile is a very saturated solution, and it has been shown that the hormones of the pill tend to make it even more saturated. In a few women this can lead to crystals separating out, followed by stone formation. The symptoms which may be caused by stones are a type of indigestion or heavy feeling in the upper part of the abdomen, particularly after meals containing a lot of fat. There may also be nausea and actual vomiting. More severe pain or jaundice may lead to hospital admission.

Apart obviously from stopping the pill, treatment can be medical or surgical. Dissolving the stones with special drugs may be successful, otherwise they are removed along with the gall-bladder. Complete recovery of full health is the rule.

The most recent research indicates that it is only early in a course of pills that there is an increased risk of gallstones. This suggests that the pill only 'brings out' an inborn tendency.

The urinary system

Cystitis and other urinary infections

Cystitis is the name for infection of the bladder. If the urine is cultured in the laboratory, a germ may be grown and the correct treatment then is an antibiotic. An increased tendency to cystitis was found among pill-users in the RCGP Study, but the Oxford/FPA Study did not find this link. This may be because the latter study looked only at infections bad enough to require referral to hospital. Even when there are no symptoms, bacteria are grown more commonly from the urine of pill-users than other women, and this would make actual infections more likely.

Women on the pill tend to have intercourse frequently, and frequent or vigorous love-making can cause cystitis – you may have heard of 'honeymoon cystitis'. Whether or not the pill is truly to blame for such infections, for some women they can be a real problem. If this is so for you, discuss the matter with your doctor. It will probably help to empty your bladder both before and after intercourse and to use a jelly lubricant (see below). You should take *plenty* of fluids – e.g. 3 litres in 3 hours – when you get an attack. Your doctor may sometimes advise taking a couple of antibiotic tablets shortly before intercourse as a regular preventive routine. Tests for vaginal infections such as thrush (page 103) may also be necessary, as these infections can cause similar symptoms. For more information see the book by Angela Kilmartin (Further reading, page 259) or ask for the Health Education Council leaflet about cystitis.

The reproductive system – (a) Gynaecology

Vaginal discharge

A few women on the pill complain of excessive dryness of the vagina. This can be quite a problem for some, and may be partly responsible for a loss of interest in sex. It can be due to the pill, usually meaning that one with relatively too high a dose of progestogen is being used (see page 178). Apart from asking about changing to another pill, it may help to have a bit more foreplay before intercourse, or occasionally to use a jelly lubricant.

However, other pill-users complain of an increase in their vaginal discharge. There are several possible causes for this:

1. *Cervical erosion*. This is a most misleading and unfortunate name for a common, quite harmless condition of the cervix. The normal covering of the outer surface of the cervix is what is known as squamous epithelium, i.e. a covering of flattened cells a little like normal skin. The normal lining of the canal that leads up into the main part of the uterus itself is columnar epithelium (upright, box-shaped cells with a lot of mucus-producing glands). All that happens if there is an erosion is that the normal lining of the canal spreads out over the outer part of the cervix. So it is not an 'ulcer', and nothing has been 'eroded' or eaten away! It just looked like that to the doctors who gave it that name, before anyone had looked at its structure under the microscope.

Erosions are about twice as common in pill-users as in non-users. The effect of having more of the type of surface which normally only lines the cervical canal is to have more mucus-producing glands: and hence an increase in the normal wetness of the vagina. Many women, pill-users or not, have this without noticing anything, but a few may call it a discharge.

All that is usually necessary is for the doctor to examine you and to take a cervical smear if you are due to have one. If, however, you are finding the amount of discharge a nuisance, perhaps requiring you to use a tampon or pad to control it, then there are very simple and painless out-patient treatments which can be arranged. After the treatment it may help to use a pill containing less of both hormones, preferably one from the bottom of a ladder in Figure 15, pages 165–7.

2. *Thrush – otherwise known as candida or monilial infection*. All three of these words apply to the same thing. It is due to a little yeast which is a very common inhabitant of the vagina, often in fact living there without causing any symptoms at all. However, it can cause an attack of intense itching of the vagina and vulva and sometimes burning on passing water, with or without a curdy, white vaginal discharge. It is more common in pregnancy; after a course of antibiotics; and in women with even very mild diabetes. Many doctors believe a small group of women may be more likely to get symptoms of the infection if they go on the pill. But surprisingly, recent research has clearly shown that the yeast itself is *not* commoner in pill-users, nor is the complaint of itching.

Anyway, if you get this trouble, it is usually easily treated with pessaries which are put into the vagina and ointment to be applied outside, all around the vulva and anus. In some women it is more troublesome, and keeps recurring. They, and also their partners, may then require extra treatments.

Trichomonas vaginitis – known as TV

There is some evidence from two British studies that this common STD (page 20), causing an itchy, fluid vaginal discharge, is *less* frequent than usual among pill-users. However, there is no proof as yet of this beneficial effect.

Pelvic infection

This also is usually due to STD and can seriously damage the uterine tubes, leading to infertility. Researchers in the USA and

103

elsewhere have found that pill-users have half the rate of this kind of infection, compared with those using no contraception. This good effect is probably due mainly to the same mucus changes in the cervix which were described on page 38, caused by progestogen. The altered mucus seems to obstruct bacteria as well as sperm. This reduces the risk of acquired infections spreading up to the womb and tubes. But it is not something to rely on – there are better ways of avoiding pelvic infection (page 19).

* Toxic-shock syndrome

This is caused by a toxin (poison) getting into the bloodstream and is produced by a bacterium, the Staphylococcus, multiplying in the vagina. The condition was recently given much publicity in the US because of its link with menstrual tampons. It is extremely rare, the more so if women change their tampons frequently. But it is dangerous, and evidence is emerging that pill-users are *less* likely to get it than others.

Ectopic pregnancy

This is the name for a pregnancy occurring in the wrong place – i.e. not in the cavity of the uterus. Described on page 192, it can lead to dangerous internal bleeding. While a woman takes the pill she is (almost) completely protected from this because she is not releasing eggs. Damaged tubes are the main cause of the problem, so she could still get an ectopic later, after stopping the pill. But there again the pill is somewhat protective because, as we have just seen, it reduces the risk of pelvic infection, and worldwide that is the main cause of tubal damage.

* Fibroids

These are lumps which can grow on the uterus. They are so common that most women get them eventually, though the size can vary from a large pinhead to as big as a football. They consist of muscle and fibrous tissue. You will probably have heard of them as an occasional cause of excessively heavy periods (menorrhagia) in some women in their late thirties or forties, who therefore require a hysterectomy (removal of the uterus). They are not cancerous. Indeed in most women no treatment at all is ever required.

How does the pill affect fibroids? Confusion reigns at present, but the news is mostly good. The RCGP Study shows that fibroids were less commonly diagnosed in pill-users. A main reason for this is probably that the heavy periods which lead to the diagnosis of fibroids if they are present simply do not happen on the pill: because the pill almost always diminishes bleeding from the uterus. Also women with fibroids tend to be less fertile, so would be less likely to go on the pill.

However, the Oxford/FPA Study did not show any effect of the pill on fibroids. To confuse the picture further, in the days of the old-fashioned high-oestrogen pills, in some individual women the fibroids were noticed to grow very rapidly if they started on the pill. This can rarely still happen today. The same sudden increase in size is sometimes seen in pregnancy, and both in pregnancy and on the pill a fibroid can suffer what is known as red degeneration. This is due to breakdown of tissue within it and causes pain.

To conclude, there is nothing to suggest the pill ever causes fibroids to appear in the first place. Some doctors believe that it might even protect users from getting them, especially if they are taking one of the more progestogen-dominant brands. Secondly, if fibroids are present, in most women the pill reduces the bleeding trouble that they may cause. But thirdly, because in a few individuals the fibroids may enlarge, women found to have them should have regular examinations as long as they stay on the pill: preferably by the same doctor each time who can notice any change in size. If available, ultrasound scan tests can also help.

Endometriosis

This is an uncommon condition which is not entirely understood but causes misery to some women. Each month they suffer from a severe aching or bruising pain before and during the period, worsened by intercourse. This is described as being different in type from menstrual cramps, though it can be just as severe. They may also have to be seen by a gynaecologist for medical or perhaps surgical treatment before they can have a baby.

It is due to some of the same kind of tissue which normally lines the uterus being present in the wrong place: such as in the ovaries (where it is one cause of cysts) or elsewhere in the reproductive system, or even further afield. How this endometrium reached these sites is often unexplained. But just as it bleeds in its correct place, in the uterus, so this wrongly situated endometrium bleeds regularly at period times; and bleeding into the tissues causes bruising pain. As in the uterus, the bleeding results from the fall in blood levels of oestrogen and progestogen.

Continuous treatment with a high-progestogen pill, or with other hormones, to abolish egg-release and therefore periods, is logical and does help if there already is endometriosis. Recently several studies have shown that this condition is also less likely to be diagnosed in the first place among women who take the pill in the ordinary way. Whether this is a genuine bonus effect of the pill has not yet been finally established.

The ovary – cysts on the ovary

Here we have another advantage of the pill: there is a certain type of ovarian cyst which can only occur in women who are not on the combined pill. These are not tumours: they are balloons containing fluid entirely surrounded by a tissue wall, developing within the ovary. They are thought to arise because of minor imbalances of the natural hormones of the menstrual cycle. Most of them start life as a follicle, stimulated to grow by FSH during the first half of the cycle as described in Chapter 2. However, instead of rupturing to release an egg, or simply losing its fluid and virtually disappearing like the other nineteen or so stimulated follicles do, the mechanism can go a bit wrong and a particular follicle can go on accumulating fluid to produce a cyst. This can be quite a big fluid-filled balloon, up to as much as 15 centimetres in size. (The egg it originally contained dies, of course, and is disposed of by the body in the normal way.) If the same thing happens over several months, several of these cysts can be produced, perhaps on each ovary. Whether single or multiple, such cysts can sometimes cause quite bad pain, including pain on intercourse. They may cure themselves (by rupturing), or rarely lead to an emergency operation – especially if the cyst causes the whole ovary on either side to twist (*torsion*).

On the pill, however, the ovaries are inactive; no follicles are stimulated to accumulate fluid; and hence things cannot go wrong so as to produce this type of cyst. Here is a way that the *combined* pill may reduce the need for surgery. (Contrast p.192.)

See also page 123 for another possible good effect of the pill on the ovary.

Effects on the cycle

See pages 176–7 for abnormalities of the bleeding pattern produced by the pill.

For most women, almost everything about periods and the so-called 'normal' cycle is improved. I say so-called 'normal' because so many women suffer some pretty annoying symptoms from their normal cycles. These can be any or all of the following: short cycles (every 3 weeks or so); irregularity; ovulation pain (Mittelschmerz); pre-menstrual tension; painful periods (dysmenorrhoea); heavy periods leading sometimes to anaemia. The 'normal' can be anything but 'nice'. If men suffered similarly, how many would agree to such a catalogue of troubles being called normal, I wonder! However, since *the pill abolishes the natural menstrual cycle altogether* (see Chapter 2), and replaces it with an apparent cycle caused simply by the fact that the pill's hormones are withdrawn for 7 days in each 28, *most of these symptoms are dramatically improved.* So much so that many women can be very reluctant to give up the pill even if they should do, perhaps, for reasons like age or smoking.

1. *Periods.* It is possible, though not normally advised (page 42), to take the ordinary combined pill continuously and then have no vaginal bleeding at all. Even if you take it in the ordinary way though, with regular breaks from pill-taking, you will notice that your 'periods' are very regular and can be accurately predicted and are usually also much lighter. As an extra bonus you are much less likely to become anaemic. This is because heavy periods can cause anaemia due to more iron (in the blood) being lost from the body than you are able to take in your diet.

If you normally suffer with *painful periods*, then the chances are also very good that these will be improved if you go on the pill. Indeed, many teenagers are put on it for this reason alone, even when they need no contraception. Period pains are caused by excessive contractions of the uterus, due mainly to substances called prostaglandins, released during the period. It seems that the thinner type of endometrium which develops in women on the pill causes less of these pain-producing substances to be released. Strangely, however, a few women, especially if underweight, actually complain of more menstrual cramping if they take some brands of pill.

2. *Mittelschmerz*. This word means 'middle pain' and refers to the pain of ovulation or egg-release. Quite a lot of women feel a slight ache in one or other groin at around the middle of the cycle, and some can use this to help them work out their 'safe period'. In some months in a few women it can be very severe. The pain is thought to be due to stretching of the rest of the ovary by the growing follicle at the middle of the cycle before it ruptures to release the egg (see Chapter 2): and when it does there may also be a small amount of painful internal bleeding. If the pain comes from the right ovary and is particularly severe, it can be very difficult to distinguish from appendicitis. Normal use of the pill prevents ovulation and so avoids both the regular monthly pain and this possibility of a mistaken diagnosis, which could even lead to an unnecessary operation.

3. *Pre-menstrual tension*. In the days leading up to the next period, many women are troubled by depression, irritability, feelings of bloatedness, weight gain, tenderness of the breasts, backache, headache, and other pains. These and other symptoms are often lumped together as the so-called 'pre-menstrual syndrome', or pre-menstrual 'tension'. Just how awful this makes this time of the month varies enormously from woman to woman, and from cycle to cycle in the same woman. But the symptoms can be quite incapacitating. It is more common for women to commit suicide, to have accidents, and to do less well than expected in exams at this time of the month than any other. Probably because the pill gives a constant dose of both types of hormone, oestrogen and progestogen, through the second half of the cycle, quite a lot of sufferers from pre-menstrual tension find it improved if they take the pill. However, some are not helped. And a few even complain of similar symptoms while taking the pill, particularly if it is a phased pill (see page 168).

4. *Ability to control the periods*. This was mentioned on page 43. It is another bonus of the pill as compared with other methods of family planning and means that if you wish you can organize when your next 'period' comes on, by simply following on with pill-taking from another packet right after the end of the current one. (For phased pills there are special rules, page 170.)

The reproductive system – (b) Fertility and babies

Return of fertility after stopping the pill

From the beginning, doctors have been aware of the possibility that the pill, which acts by suppressing the normal menstrual cycle, might delay its normal return. This might interfere with the ability of ex-pill-users to have babies when they wanted them. The Oxford/FPA Study was reassuring. Among previously fertile women giving up contraception so as to conceive, by about 30 months those who stopped the pill were as likely to have had their next baby as ex-users of the IUD or the cap. But it does seem from this and the RCGP Study that ex-pill-users take about three months longer to conceive than ex-users of other methods – ON AVERAGE. No one knows in advance how fertile a particular relationship will be; and it is important to remember that some women can get pregnant while using the pill just because they forget one or two tablets!

There is a substantial minority of 10 to 15 per cent of women who, whatever previous method of family planning they have used, fail to get pregnant after trying for a baby for a year. This is the proportion of reduced fertility which is to be expected in any community. So if a woman stops the pill and fails to get pregnant, although it is very natural to blame the pill there is a better than one in ten chance that it could be a coincidence.

Fertility also goes down with age. So sometimes the problem is partly connected with delaying too long before trying for a baby. This is a most important point. All methods of family planning share a common 'side-effect': they give modern women the freedom to delay starting their family, but this can sometimes be for a bit too long. Some women suffer from infertility at 35, yet could have conceived without difficulty at 20. Indeed a few have proved that by an earlier unplanned pregnancy. If possible, try to start your family in your twenties or early thirties.

A very few women, perhaps 1 in 200 who stop the pill, develop amenorrhoea – absence of ovulation and of periods – for over six months. Experts believe that in only a few such cases was the pill responsible, and even then only bringing out a natural tendency. Usually the previous pill-use was a coincidence, and the regular *substitute* periods they were having on the pill were masking amenorrhoea. It has not been linked with any particular brand, and can happen if the pill was used briefly or for a long time. So there is no logic in taking a routine break every two years on fertility grounds. Reassuringly, it is now also possible to treat this problem with almost 100 per cent success. (See also pages 63 and 158.)

Perhaps we should turn the figures round and point out that in about 999 out of 1,000 women the pill method is entirely reversible, and that on stopping it they get back the fertility that nature gave them – *for the age that they have now reached.*

Please note too that the problem of absent periods *after* stopping, or without ever having taken, the pill is a completely different one from absence of 'pill periods'. The latter means nothing at all in relation to your chances of having a baby in the future. In fact, those few women who have absent periods after stopping the pill very commonly had very regular 'periods' – hormone withdrawal bleeds – all the time that they were taking it. See pages 39, 176–7 for further discussion of this matter which many people find confusing.

Could the pill cause my next baby to be abnormal?

1. *After stopping the pill?* Provided it was discontinued well before conceiving, researchers have failed to detect any consistent increase – or decrease – in any type of abnormality. In 1980 there was a report about what are known as neural tube defects, or NTDs, (a group of birth defects which include spina bifida). It appeared that in South Wales there was an increased rate of NTDs among the offspring of women who conceived within three months of stopping the pill.

Researchers from South Wales and Leeds have also reported that if a woman had had a *previous* NTD baby, the risk of having another could be reduced if she took extra vitamins before and after the time of conception. If this means that NTDs are in part caused by low vitamin levels, and we know (page 73) that the pill lowers many of these, an ex-use effect of the pill looks possible.

All the same, other studies, before and since, especially a large one from Finland in 1981, have quite failed to show any link between NTDs and recent use of the pill. Moreover an expert Scientific Group of the World Health Organization (WHO) declared in 1981 that there was no evidence for any adverse effects on the fetus of pill-use prior to conception. Twin-births seem to be less common, however.

What then should you do if you are on the pill and want to stop it for a baby? All couples are advised to delay conception at least until after the first *natural* period (see page 63). Those couples who are by nature extra cautious may, in addition, use a method like the sheath to arrange that three months go by before their planned baby is conceived. This has not been proved to help, though it should certainly do no harm. On the whole it is better only to take extra vitamins in tablet form, either at this time or after conception, if so advised by your doctor. According to some of the research, the most relevant vitamin is probably *folic acid*, but there is plenty of this in any balanced diet. Good food sources include green vegetables, citrus fruits, lean meats, liver, kidney and yeast extracts. All the researchers agree that a good diet is in fact the main thing.

Most importantly, any woman who finds herself pregnant less than three months after stopping the pill should not be alarmed. Literally millions of mothers have done this without any harm befalling their babies. The extra risk of NTDs is unproven, and if it exists it is clearly very, very small. If in doubt or anxious about this matter, make sure you discuss it with your doctor. Depending on your particular circumstances and all the pros and cons involved, certain tests which should reliably rule out most types of NTD can now be done during early pregnancy.

2. *What about pill-taking in early pregnancy?* The RCGP Study researchers have reported that 102 babies were born following pregnancies during which the pill continued to be taken for a while, usually by mistake. In the Oxford/FPA Study there were a further 66 such births. The rate of birth defects in these was no higher than would be expected in any group of women having a planned baby. But it seems that in these circumstances twinning is more likely (contrast with page 110).

This is most reassuring. Although 168 babies is not an enormous number, it must mean that *any adverse effect on unborn babies of the hormones used in current pills must be very infrequent*. However, we cannot leave the story there. The articles published about unplanned pregnancy while taking the pill are many, but they are also contradictory and very confusing. To summarize things very briefly, it does seem that the high-dose artificial sex hormones which used to be taken by women to help to make the diagnosis of pregnancy could perhaps harm the baby. But now that there are perfectly safe and more accurate methods based on measuring the hormone hCG (page 29) in a sample of early morning urine, this outdated way of testing for pregnancy should never be used at all. These hormone pregnancy tests were rather different from the combined pill anyway, as they used much higher doses. Secondly, you may perhaps have heard the very disquieting story of the drug diethylstilboestrol (DES). This is even less relevant to the pill, as this variety of oestrogen – which has a quite different chemical formula – *never has been and never will be used in any combined contraceptive pills*. But the story does worry some people about the pill, so let us discuss it and learn its lessons here.

Shortly after the last war there was a vogue, particularly in America, to treat threatened miscarriage with DES, a synthetic oestrogen. It was later shown that the treatment made no difference to the outcome when bleeding occurred in early pregnancy. But the doctors concerned thought that at least no harm had been done to those babies who were born if the pregnancies did not miscarry. Tragically, however, although the girl babies who were born in these circumstances appeared entirely normal at birth, they proved much later on – as teenagers – to be more likely to develop a form of cancer of the vagina that was previously almost unknown. If their mothers had been treated with this drug in pregnancy about one in a thousand of these girls got this cancer. Other problems in the daughters, and even in the mothers, have been suggested by some researchers. Boys born following pregnancies treated with DES were also reported to be more likely to have various abnormalities of their urinary system or genital organs.

This sad story rams home the message, once again, that all except life-saving or proven safe drug treatment should be avoided during early pregnancy, particularly during the crucial first three months while all the organs of the baby are being formed.

What does this mean in practice? Even though there is no proof that the pill could harm a baby, it is surely best to play safe. You should never *start* taking contraceptives or any other hormones if you think you could already be pregnant. And if you think you might have become pregnant while taking the combined or progestogen-only pill, it is best to switch at once to another

112

method until you know for sure one way or another. This is discussed in relation to missed or not-absorbed pills in Figures 11 (page 50) and 18 (page 188).

If pregnancy is confirmed, and you did take pills *after the conception*, it is you who must decide what, if anything, to do; though consultation with your partner and the doctor may help. Discuss whether any special tests should be done, such as those mentioned earlier (page 111). The increased risk of an abnormality must be very small indeed, judging by those 168 babies mentioned earlier. This was also the view of that WHO Scientific Group (page 110). One estimate, which I think could well be an overestimate, is *less than* one in a thousand: this was based mainly on babies born to mothers who took hormones other than for contraception, including the high dose of hormones for pregnancy testing. Moreover, that figure should be compared with the fact – surprising to most people – that 1 in 50 of all babies have a serious birth defect.

The breasts

Breast enlargement

Some women say their breasts seem smaller, but far more users of the pill do notice their bust getting a little larger. The increase tends to reach its maximum by the second packet of pills, and not to continue afterwards. For most women and their partners, and in most cultures, this is seen as an advantage. Others may object. It occurs partly as a direct effect of the progestogen and oestrogen, but also because many pill-users have an increase in the blood level of one of their own hormones, prolactin. This is produced by the pituitary gland, and one of its effects is to stimulate the breasts.

* In fact, prolactin can occasionally do rather too good a job of breast stimulation, and lead to:

The appearance of milky fluid from the nipples

This unwanted secretion can be a nuisance and should always be mentioned to your doctor. This is because the level of the hormone prolactin ought to be measured, as, if it is particularly high, it could perhaps be coming from a pituitary adenoma. This is a 'tiny lump', sometimes microscopic in size, formed in the

113

pituitary gland. Such lumps can be treated very satisfactorily either medically or, rarely, by an operation. The pill is not thought to cause them but, like pregnancy, it could make them enlarge and become more active if present. So if the pill is used at all in this rare condition, it should only be under expert supervision.

Tenderness of the breasts

This can be part of the whole range of symptoms of pre-menstrual tension, or it can occur alone. In some unfortunate women the tenderness can be so extreme that for a few days before each period they cannot bear their breasts being touched, even by clothing. If you have this problem (even if not quite as bad as that) you may be better off while on the pill. It is possible that you will not be helped; and a few women actually report the symptom for the first time on the pill, especially during the early months. There is an enormous amount of variation in how people respond to drugs, and the pill is no exception to that rule.

Benign breast disease

This general term is used to include a number of non-malignant problems of the breast which are sometimes called 'chronic mastitis', 'fibrocystic disease', and a variety of other names. They all refer to more or less generalized lumpiness of the breast which can be quite tender and vary from month to month and with the time of the month, usually worst just before a period. This is a definite plus point for the pill, as the commonest microscopic type of this breast trouble tends to be much less common during pill-use, especially long-term pill-use. Some-times there is a definite lump which no surgeon can be sure is not cancer till he has removed it, and had it looked at under a microscope by a laboratory expert. As a result, quite often women have to be admitted for an operation, under general anaesthesia, to remove what is actually a benign breast lump. Yet this is the only safe way to handle the situation. The point is that this chain of events is less likely in any woman who uses the pill. Here then is another kind of surgical operation that is statistically less likely if you are on the pill, which for this effect should be a fixed-dose type and preferably progestogen dominant (page 132). If you have had breast surgery, see page 121.

Interference with breast-feeding

The combined pill can quite commonly reduce the volume and quality of milk flow in women who are breast-feeding after recently having had a baby. It seems pointless to use the combined pill at this time, when the progestogen-only pill is available which does not interfere with the flow of milk (see Chapter 8). In combination with full breast-feeding the progestogen-only pill is close to 100 per cent effective.

Bones and joints

*Premature closing of the epiphyses

There is a theoretical effect of oestrogen in the pill, that it might stop a young girl growing before she had achieved her full height. This is because oestrogen can affect the epiphyses (growing-points) of the long bones, to cause them to close prematurely. It is considered most unlikely, however, that this would happen in practice with the tiny dose of oestrogen in modern pills, and following the normal rules: i.e. the pill should never be given until, at the earliest, menstrual cycles have become well and truly established. See also page 67 for other important considerations; and pages 120–1, 129 for the reasons why it is prudent to use the lowest acceptable dose in this age-group, especially of the progestogen hormone.

* Arthritis

Recent research has suggested that women on the pill are less likely to suffer from one common and troublesome variety known as rheumatoid arthritis. If this protection effect turns out to be true it can only be quite small. Out of every 3,000 pill-users only 1 per year who would otherwise get the disease will avoid it. However, if she knew this was so she would undoubtedly be grateful! See also page 118.

The skin

Chloasma/melasma

These unusual words describe a fairly common brown discoloration which is mainly on the forehead and on each side of the face in front of the ears. It is obviously not a problem for black-skinned women, but can happen to other races in pregnancy (the 'pregnancy mask'), and to pill-users. It is usually first noticed when the weather is good. Some women also notice an increase of pigmentation in other parts of the body. Special sunscreen creams can be applied especially during the summer, and careful use of make-up when required may help.

Chloasma usually fades a little when the pill is stopped or, apparently, after transferring to the progestogen-only pill. It may not entirely disappear though, because of pigment having been actually laid down in the skin.

Photosensitivity (excessive sensitivity to sunlight)

This problem can affect women who have never been on the pill, but it is about four times more common in those who have. Skin exposed to the sun's rays develops very itchy red weals or 'hives' (urticaria). Treatment for this is unsatisfactory and there may be only a slight improvement if the pill is stopped. It is fairly uncommon, but it may mean that the affected woman has to avoid sunbathing altogether. Very rarely it is an indication of one of the porphyrias (page 152).

＊ *Increase in facial or body hair (hirsutism)*

This is fortunately very rare, especially with the modern low-dose pills, and sometimes may be a coincidence. Changing to an oestrogen-dominant pill may help (page 178) and is well worth trying before giving the method up altogether. These pills can be such a help that they are sometimes recommended to treat people with excessive hair growth who have no need of the pill for contraception. Extra hair may also have to be removed with the help of electrolysis or similar treatment from a skin specialist.

＊ *Loss of scalp hair*

This can also occur in women who have never taken any sex hormones at all. In fact there was no suggestion in the RCGP Study that this might be caused by the pill. Like after childbirth, however, it is reported that some women have a problem of excessive hair loss *after* stopping the pill. This corrects itself spontaneously, though full recovery of decent-length head hair could take a year or more.

116

A range of other skin troubles has been described, occurring for the first time or apparently being worsened in pill-users. Yet others are improved. They tend to have rather complicated names. Out of a long list, those which are probably or possibly promoted by the pill include: telangiectasia, rosacea, eczema, neurodermatitis, erythema nodosum, and erythema multiforme. Some of these may be linked to the problem of allergy (see page 118 for further discussion). Herpes gestationis is another one, interesting because, like the form of jaundice mentioned on page 100, it can occur in pregnancy and is likely to recur or worsen if the same woman later goes on the pill.

Even added together these skin troubles are still quite uncommon. Rather than say more about them here, *from the practical point of view* you should take advice from your doctor if you ever develop any skin problem which you think might be due to or made worse by the pill.

Skin troubles often made better by the pill

1. *Acne*. The RCGP Study showed that this was particularly likely to be improved, but at the time all pills had 50 micrograms or more of oestrogen in them. The story now seems a bit more complicated. Acne occurs chiefly because the tiny ducts or passages leading from the grease-producing glands of the skin, especially in the face and on the back, tend to get blocked. The oestrogen in the pill may help to stop this happening. Some women are simply unlucky in the actual grease-producing glands they have been given by nature, and just going on the pill may not be enough to help the situation. However, if your own acne is not improved or seems to be getting worse on the pill, it may be worth asking to change to a more oestrogen-dominant brand (see pages 178–9). There are also other treatments, and fortunately the problem does tend to improve with age.

2. *Hirsutism*. Oestrogen-dominant pills can sometimes help this problem of unwanted hair growth too (pages 178–9).

3. *Greasy hair*. This too may be helped by oestrogen-dominant pills.

4. *Wax in the ears*. The wax-producing glands of the ears are affected in rather the same way by the hormones of the pill as the grease-producing glands. As a result the RCGP Study also

showed that you were less likely to have to have your ears syringed for wax in them if you were on the pills then in use!

* Anything else?

On top of everything mentioned elsewhere in these two chapters, the evidence is becoming stronger for most of the following collection of possible side-effects: the carpal tunnel syndrome, in which there is a *gradual* onset of tingling and pain in one or both hands; cramps and pains in the legs; gingivitis (inflammation of the gums); dry socket after tooth extraction; vertigo (dizziness); voice changes in singers; Raynaud's syndrome (excessive whitening and 'deadness' of the fingers in cold weather); and chilblains.

I have left till now two very important but more general subjects, about which there are at the present time more questions than answers.

* The body's immunity and allergy mechanisms

The RCGP, Oxford/FPA and Walnut Creek Studies all showed that pill-users were more likely than non-users to have various infections including chicken pox, gastric flu, respiratory and urinary infections. There is also a suggestion from some sources that the pill might reduce resistance to malaria, though not by enough to discourage its use in malarious areas.

Other inflammations, of soft tissues or of the bowel (tenosynovitis, bursitis, synovitis, ulcerative colitis, and Crohn's disease) have also been reported more commonly in pill-users.

These facts suggest that the pill can alter *immunity*. In addition, various skin troubles are often connected with *allergy*, and eczema, for instance, was twice as common in pill-users in the RCGP Study. Women can also develop an allergy, with specific antibodies (see page 208 for a further explanation of these), to either the progestogen or the oestrogen of the pill itself. This occurs more rarely than with other commonly used drugs like penicillins, but can show itself by troublesome rashes or by painful swollen joints (polyarthritis). These clear up completely only when the pill is stopped, and would recur if the same hormone were to be given again. So allergies to the pill itself certainly occur. Whether allergies to other substances happen more readily because the pill is being taken is not so clear, though the increased rate of hay fever is suggestive (page 99).

Another possibility is allergy to a person's own tissues causing so-called *auto-immune diseases*. It does appear that the pill can sometimes aggravate the symptoms and signs of one of these, systemic lupus erythematosus (SLE), which affects connective tissues in the body.

The number of white cells in the blood is increased in pill-users, and experiments on those called lymphocytes – which are much involved in this immune/allergy system – have shown that the pill can alter their activities.

The immune/allergy system is involved in causing several types of thyroid disease and also rheumatoid arthritis. As the pill seems to protect against these diseases (pages 75 and 115), perhaps these good effects too are due to an alteration in this system, caused by the pill's hormones.

What about cancer?

The pill does contain powerful hormones, and hormones have been shown to affect the growth of some cancers, in animals and in humans. So ever since the pill was first marketed there has always been the possibility that it might be found to increase the risk of some type of cancer. Secondly, it is one of the best-known facts of cancer research that cancers may not develop until after many years – up to thirty years – of exposure to any cancer-producing agent. The pill has been around for only about twenty years. We are therefore only now beginning to obtain useful information about possible links between the pill and some forms of cancer. Although in most cases these have not yet been confirmed, in view of the widespread nature of the pill's effects we should not be too surprised if it can in fact modify the risk of getting certain cancers. The important thing is that it could operate either way: promoting some but actually reducing the likelihood of other types. Two examples of cancers which are *less* frequent in pill-takers than other women are those which start in the endometrium and the ovary (see below).

So it begins to look a bit like 'swings and roundabouts', with the good effects tending to balance the bad, and the *overall* risk of cancer staying about the same as that for the general population. But this is an unfolding story, which will not be fully told for some time yet.

* The breast

In the United States, it seems that one in every 11 women will develop breast cancer at some time in her life. Many will eventually die, years later, of something quite different. And the rate is not quite so high in other developed countries, such as Britain. But if the pill were found to cause any change in the frequency of this disease – either way – it would be enormously important.

During the last 25 years the pill has increasingly been used, and breast-cancer rates have increased in many countries. It is tempting to conclude that the pill is to blame. If that were so, it is odd that the statistics show a rise in all age-groups, and the greatest rise among the older women who never took the pill. Moreover there have been many other relevant changes in the same 25 years: in diet for a start, plus increased rates of several known risk factors. These include:

- Younger ages at the first menstrual period.
- Later ages at the menopause.
- More women delaying the birth of their first child. (This is known to increase breast-cancer rates whatever method of family planning is used.)
- The family history of a close relative with breast cancer.

Unhelpfully, the research in this field is complicated, confusing, and often contradictory. Until October 1983 there was good general agreement that the evidence did not support a link between the pill and this cancer. The biggest study in the USA, known as the CASH (Cancer and Steroid Hormones) Study, reassuringly found somewhat *fewer* pill-takers among the cancer patients than among the matched comparison women with no cancer. Several studies have also shown that pill-takers tend to have their cancer diagnosed at an earlier stage and to have a better outlook following treatment.

Then in October and December 1983 there were two reports in the journal the *Lancet* which caused a new concern. Could the pill increase the risk for a particular group, those who used it for a long time either under age 25, or maybe prior to the delivery of their first baby? These reports, one by Dr Pike from the USA and the other from Britain, have been criticized on many counts (to do with the methods used), but suggested a three or four times increased risk if the pill were so used for more than four years.

However, the CASH Study includes more cases than the above studies had between them. By the end of 1983 the researchers had details of 700 young women with breast cancer and a matched group without the disease, and could show no difference between them in pill usage either before age 25 or before their first baby!

What now, in practice? Despite conflicting information, there is the good news that even in the Pike Study there was a group of pills which seemed to be free of blame, namely those whose progestogen content – or rather its biological activity – was low. So while we wait for more research we should surely choose from this group, and select those brands which are also low in oestrogen so as to minimize the blood-clotting risks. This policy is strongly supported on other grounds too, for older women as well as those under 25; see pages 131–3, 172–5.

Secondly, whether or not they have ever taken the pill, and especially if any of the above risk factors apply, *all women should examine their own breasts regularly* each month. This is best done after periods, using the flat of the extended fingers. This is just common sense, and if you are in any doubt about how to do it you should ask to be taught by your doctor or nurse, with the help of an illustrated leaflet – see page 264.

If you are seeing a surgeon for a problem with your breasts, take his expert advice as to whether he feels it advisable to continue with or start taking the pill. The decision depends on the precise microscopic appearances of any part of the breast that has been looked at in the laboratory. The family history is always important (see above, and page 160). But if a woman actually has had breast cancer treated, she should stop or avoid the pill and all sex hormones except as part of treatment recommended by the doctor looking after her for the disease.

The uterus – (a) the cervix (entrance to the womb)

Here is another change from the last edition. A new report in 1983 from the Oxford/FPA Study (page 87) suggests increased rates of this cancer, and of the pre-cancer changes picked up by cervical smears, with increasing duration of use of the pill. After more than eight years the maximum rate was 2–3 times that in non-users (actually IUD-users). Another researcher also reported in 1977 that the pill seemed to accelerate the slow rate at which the earliest changes can sometimes progress to actual cancer, though other workers have not found this effect.

Cancer of the cervix is really a sexually transmitted disease (page 21). It is caused either by a virus or some chemical carried by sperm to the cervix. Hence barrier methods like the diaphragm are protective. The risk for someone with many sexual partners can be hundreds of times that for a one-man woman whose partner is a one-woman man. This much exceeds the pill effect, even if we accept the Oxford report – which needs to be confirmed by other good studies (always important, see page 88).

In practice, the main point is that pill-users should have regular cervical smears. How often? This is another disputed point, but the main factor is your own sex life (page 21).

Secondly, *take your doctor's advice if you have actually had an abnormal smear.* Mild changes commonly resolve naturally, so the smear may just be repeated every few months. Or the abnormality may have been removed by minor surgery. Some doctors now feel that either of these situations is a *relative contra-indication* (page 160). But my present view is that if after full discussion of all the facts, and the question marks, you prefer the pill to any of the alternatives, your choice should be respected. Frequent smears as ordered by your gynaecologist will of course be vital, while on the pill and probably for the rest of your life.

(b) The endometrium (lining of the womb)

Cancer of this type was more likely to occur in women who used the high-oestrogen so-called 'sequential' pills. (These are no longer prescribed for contraception.) But the complete opposite applies to ordinary combined pills. The CASH researchers (see

122

page 120) have shown a *halving* of the risk if the pill is taken for at least one year, and a threefold reduction after five years. This protective effect has been confirmed by at least six other studies, and encouragingly seems to persist in ex-users – for ten years, possibly even longer.

* *The ovary*

At least nine studies report a clear-cut protective effect against this particularly fatal type of cancer, which is greater the longer the pill has been used. After five years there is a two to threefold reduction in the risk, and once again some protection continues among ex-users for at least ten years, maybe even for life.

It is probably not coincidental that both the last two cancers are beneficially affected by the pill: both are commoner in those women who have had many menstrual cycles, an unnatural state of affairs which is avoided by pill-takers. See pages 40–1.

* *Hydatidiform mole*

There is no simpler name for this strange condition in which there is complete failure of the normal development of a pregnancy. It is not itself a cancer, but it has a very small risk of turning into one. No embryo develops, and the afterbirth fills the uterus to make it seem like a bag full of very mushy grapes. These produce large amounts of the special pregnancy hormone hCG (see page 29). Sooner or later, as this is never going to be a successful pregnancy, bleeding occurs. Eventually the uterus has to be emptied under anaesthetic in hospital, by a D & C.

Subsequently, the patient has to be very carefully followed up. The main thing that has to be done during follow-up is a regular special blood or urine test to measure the hCG level. In Britain these tests are mailed to specified Regional Centres. In nearly all patients, the level falls steadily to nil in a few months, and that is really the end of the story. In a *tiny* minority, however, the level of hCG stays up, and this means that powerful drugs must be given as it is due to the very beginnings of a cancer called choriocarcinoma. If this is treated early the outcome is almost always complete cure.

The pill does not make the original hydatidiform mole more likely to happen, but it comes into the story here. Researchers in London have shown that if the pill is taken before the hCG level

123

in the blood has declined to zero, the chances of needing the powerful drug treatment for the early cancer are about doubled. Other research workers have failed to confirm this, however.

Until the uncertainty is resolved, in my view, both combined and progestogen-only pills are best avoided altogether by a woman who has had this unusual trouble – but only until she is informed that her hCG test is back to normal. After discussion with her gynaecologist or other doctor, oral contraception could then be considered once again as an option.

*Melanoma

This cancer can develop from a mole of a quite different kind, one of the black patches which people have on their skin. Almost everyone has a few of these. But they very rarely become cancerous, particularly in Britain, as this change seems to be more likely in skin exposed to a lot of sunlight. In areas like California and Australia where there is a lot of sun it seemed possible in some studies, but not in others, that the pill might slightly increase the chances of the transformation of an ordinary mole into this cancer. But as there is a possibility that pill-users in the research populations may have sunbathed more than non-users, there is no proof yet that the pill directly promotes this rare cancer.

*Liver

There is a hint but no proof that the pill may promote primary cancer of the liver, an exceedingly rare disease. Tumours of a non-cancerous kind are more certainly linked with long-term use, though they too are very rare. They appear as lumps on the liver, and as they contain a great many blood-vessels they can sometimes cause dangerous internal bleeding – leading to an emergency operation to stop this and remove the tumour.

To conclude, if all the 'pros' and 'cons' are carefully weighed up, the evidence so far does not disprove the following statement:

The average informed pill-user may continue to take modern ultra-low-dose pills without fearing any increase in her OVERALL cancer risk.

How long should she continue? See pages 126–30. And remember, the situation is constantly under review, as new facts emerge.

* How reliable are the research studies on the pill?

Although they are the best available, we do have to be a little cautious when applying the results of research like the RCGP, Walnut Creek and Oxford/FPA Studies. For a start, there are differences between the sort of women who use a method like the pill and those who do not. These differences could lead to any trouble or apparent benefit which arises being put down to the pill when it was really connected with some other feature of the woman herself. In general, pill-users seem to be generally healthier than non-users, rather than the reverse.

Secondly, in the RCGP and Walnut Creek Studies, though not in the Oxford/FPA one, the pill-users went more often to their doctors as a routine, to collect their prescriptions. While there, they could be more likely to mention a problem they had noticed than the non-pill-users with whom they were compared, who would have to make a special visit. As the research workers are aware of this possible bias attempts have been made to allow for it.

Thirdly, most studies omit teenagers, and use of *modern* pills (page 142).

What about the risks of the pill in less developed countries?

These have been inadequately examined so far. The research has nearly all been done in 'over-developed' countries, where diseases of the circulation such as heart attacks and strokes in relatively young people are commoner than in developing countries. This is probably because there are so many things wrong with the diet, combined with the popularity of smoking and the unpopularity of exercise, among other things. This would suggest that use of the pill should be even more reasonable for women in the less developed countries; particularly in comparison with the tragically high rate of death and serious complications of pregnancy and childbirth in the absence of good medical care, which many of them have to face (see Figure 1).

A special advantage of the pill is connected with anaemia of the type due to shortage of iron, which is more common because of malnutrition and conditions such as worms. The pill reduces both blood loss at 'periods' and loss of iron to the baby in repeated pregnancies. On the other hand, the pill has effects on vitamins (see Table 3 on page 72, and page 75). Recent research suggests that extra vitamins are helpful for women with dietary deficiencies – but *not* for healthy pill-users anywhere.

Research in developing countries by international bodies such as the World Health Organization (WHO) is now showing some differences in body chemistry. Pill-users in Dublin get more of the changes favouring blood-clotting than women in Salvador (Brazil) taking the same brand. And, according to some researchers, poor nutrition and reduced amounts of body fat may lower the blood levels of the pill's hormones after taking standard pills. Thus, underweight, malnourished women may, paradoxically, be at extra risk of pregnancy, and probably should not take the very lowest-dose pills. Another factor which favours slightly higher-dose pills is the observation that erratic pill-taking is rather common among women in developing countries (depending very much on how well they have been taught).

We just do not know how important differences between women in the less developed countries and those who have been studied in the 'over-developed' world may be. Differences might be expected due to heredity: for example, there could be as yet undiscovered racial differences in body chemistry, leading to different handling of the pill's hormones by the body. The effects that being on the pill might have in women suffering from the various chronic tropical diseases are still being studied, including: malaria (see page 118); leprosy; liver fluke infection; and bilharzia. WHO has reported a possible slight increase in activity of the parasites among pill-users with bilharzia. But the pill had no harmful effects on tests of liver function in this disease.

More research is needed. But so far no reports have identified any definite extra risk for pill-users in developing countries compared with those in Europe and North America.

What are the long-term or long-delayed effects of taking the pill?

For an individual woman, this question needs to be broken down to three different but closely connected questions:

1. *How long should one continue taking the pill?*
2. *Should one take breaks* every two years or every five years?
3. Irrespective of the answers to questions 1 and 2, *what is the upper age limit for continuing to take the pill?*

126

From the point of view of preserving *future fertility*, the answer is clear to all these questions. There is no connection between fertility problems and how long the pill was previously used, in total, with or without breaks. Routine breaks at any set time interval are therefore illogical (page 110). The combined pill seems to be truly a reversible method of contraception. And the upper age limit for the best chance of success when it comes to trying for a baby is the same, whether discontinuing the pill or any other method. If circumstances permit, try to start your family in your twenties or early thirties.

* Side-effects

Most of the risks (and benefits) seem to apply only while the pill is actually being taken. And if the pill is stopped, things seem to return to normal within a few weeks. These statements apply to the studies of body chemistry which were described earlier (page 75, and Table 3, page 72); to the risk of many of the serious side-effects such as venous thrombosis, and of the less serious but annoying ones such as weight gain and headaches; and of course to the beneficial effects on the menstrual cycle.

As a general rule, for most good and bad effects, there is no evidence of their being enhanced or increased in frequency by increasing duration of use if that factor is considered independently of age; nor of persistence in ex-users. However, there are some exceptions to this general statement. For example, if the pill promotes allergy (page 118) – something that has not yet been proved – any allergy that developed would tend to persist for the rest of the life of that individual. A discussion of some other possible exceptions follows below.

* Diseases of the circulation

As stated on page 88, the RCGP Study now shows no detectable increase in the overall risk with increasing duration of use in current users. However, in a later report (1983), the researchers were more doubtful about the absence of a duration-of-use effect for individual diseases, particularly stroke. It has also been shown before that raised blood pressure is diagnosed increasingly often, the longer the pill has been used. These remain the only two exceptions – no duration-of-use effect has yet been found for other conditions such as heart attack or venous thrombosis.

* *Possible residual effects in ex-users*

The increased risk of strokes does appear from the latest RCGP research to continue in ex-users, for more than six years after the pill was last taken. Although this is disturbing, it is important to remember that strokes are extremely rare in young women; the risk appears to be focused on those with other risk factors (pages 81–2), especially smoking; and it is probably also at a lower level than in current users.

Another study from the USA, has shown an ex-use effect of the pill on coronary thrombosis. It was found that ex-users of the pill over the age of 40 were about twice as likely to suffer a heart attack as comparable never-users. But this was only if the ex-users had used the pill for more than five years in the past, and mainly in heavy smokers who used the pill in their thirties, which is not now advised. This study also raised a new question. Among ex-users, especially smokers, could such a residual effect on the heart-attack risk be greater the longer they *previously* took the pill? The possibility is there, in their data, but it seems somewhat unlikely given the absence (mentioned above) of a duration-of-use effect in current users!

How then do we minimize the risk of diseases of the circulation?

Age? This question among those which began this section was really answered on pages 90–1. Smokers should consider stopping at age 30 and must transfer to another method at the age of 35. For non-smokers without other risk factors, the normal upper limit is set at 40 years, though in my view it is permissible for some women to continue using it up to age 45. This would only be at their insistence and after the most careful assessment of their total situation, coupled as appropriate with special blood tests (perhaps a blood-group test – page 82; test for blood fats – page 132; and if relevant a Glucose Tolerance Test – page 74). Such women should also have their blood pressure measured at least every 6 months.

Breaks? We can, I think, give the answer 'no' to the question about taking breaks every two or every five years. Even if one takes action on the most worrying evidence available (which is disputed), there is nothing to suggest that taking breaks would reduce the risk, unless these were long enough to have a definite impact on the total accumulated duration of use. In other words, suppose a pill-user decides to take a six-month break every two years: after twelve years she will have accumulated ten years of use, without, so far as we know, lessening her risk as compared with someone who took the pill continuously for ten years. In short, *repeated breaks from pill-taking are a nuisance, are of no proven benefit, and also have been known to lead to unplanned pregnancies* . . .

Duration? While we wait for further information about residual effects, it seems to me prudent to set some limits on total duration of use. The issue might first be faced after ten years' accumulated use (with or without breaks). Smokers should consider 15 years as the absolute maximum, provided they are also under 35 and have normal blood pressure. Non-smokers under 45 who are free of risk factors might be given, at their request, an upper limit of 20 years' use.

Cancer and duration of use/ex-use

Please read pages 119–24, if you have not already done so. If the pill is finally proved to increase the risk of any cancer – not so, as yet – the harmful effect could be greater the longer the pill were used, and might persist to some extent in ex-users. If the pill reduces a risk, as it does for cancer of the ovary and endometrium, the protective effect is likewise greater the longer the duration of use, and continues among ex-users.

Once again – see page 120 – we have 'swings and round-abouts': good effects of long-term pill-use tending to balance the bad. For the present the above rules for minimizing circulatory-disease risk are also good working rules for cancer risk. As before, breaks are unlikely to help as the evidence points to total duration. But in this context there are more question marks about long-term use by *the young*. So far the evidence about breast cancer (page 120) does not support setting an arbitrary limit to the number of years' use by women under age 25 or before their first baby – unless they are at special risk (page 160).

In conclusion, nothing stated here overrides the importance of your own views and intuition. By all means take short-term or longer breaks if this helps your own peace of mind. But do be careful in your use of another method, without gambling! – unless you really want a baby.

* What do the changes in body chemistry mean?

See Table 3 (page 72). A wide variety of changes have been described in the blood of pill-users, and often their meaning from the point of view of the health of the person concerned is completely unknown. Some of them must be connected in some way with known unwanted effects of the pill: for instance, the changes in blood lipids and clotting factors. Even here the full details of the connection between the blood changes and the appearance of symptoms are not fully worked out. The majority of the remainder seem harmless, but only time and a lot more research will prove if this is so.

One of the main aims of research into body chemistry is to find a simple and accurate test of a body fluid such as blood or, preferably, saliva or urine, which would identify those women who should *not* be on the pill because they are at too high a risk of trouble. A lot can already be done to avoid giving the pill to women at special risk (see page 149). Tests on blood and other fluids, however, have so far been disappointing; blood lipid (fat) studies are very complicated and even the experts may not be sure what they mean in any individual. They are not suitable as so-called 'screening' tests and have to be reserved primarily for women who have a family history suggesting that they might prove to be abnormal. None of the tests of various clotting factors, of which there are very many, has yet been found to give a practical 'alarm signal' that a particular woman should avoid or discontinue the pill. This is the kind of test we need: but it also must be very cheap and easy to use in field conditions if it is to be any help in the less developed countries.

Of course, there is already one quite useful test: the blood pressure of pill-users. Stopping the pill when this becomes raised may prevent a stroke from occurring (page 84) and *may* perhaps protect the pill-user from other troubles too (page 86).

Are there differences between the different brands of pill?

The short answer is 'yes, but we do not know in detail what they are'. There are over thirty different varieties of pill, including progestogen-only pills, on the British market, and other formulations are also used in other countries. Two different oestrogens are used and several different progestogens, in varying combinations. The currently available British ones are shown in Tables 8, 9 and 11 (pages 162, 163, 194). As the next section explains, low-dose brands from Table 8 are now preferred. They all use the same oestrogen (ethinyloestradiol), but it is impossible to say which progestogen is 'the best buy'. All we can say at present is that the first-choice pill for a new user would usually be one giving the lowest available dose of *both* hormones (see page 175).

* How much safer are the modern very low-oestrogen pills? and the progestogen-only pills?

Although we cannot distinguish between individual brands, research is available that strongly suggests that, as far as risk is concerned, the lower the dose of artificial hormone taken, the better: and the amount of hormones in pills taken for contraception has diminished most dramatically since they were first introduced. Table 5 shows how in the modern ultra-low-dose combined pills, which are still highly effective against pregnancy, it is possible to use more than seven times less oestrogen in one

Table 5 Reduction in hormone dose given since combined pills were first introduced

	Amount used then (1960–2)	*Minimum* of same hormone used now (1984)
Dose (micrograms) of oestrogen (ethinyloestradiol)	150 mcg in Enovid 10	20 mcg in Loestrin 20
Dose (milligrams) of progestogen (norethisterone)	10 mg in Ortho-novum 10	0.5 mg in { Ovysmen { Brevinor

pill and twenty times less progestogen in another pill than were used in varieties that were first introduced in the early 1960s. It seems now that the old idea that oestrogen was the main hormone causing unwanted effects is too simple. *Oestrogen* is certainly the hormone that causes the main changes in clotting factors, predisposing to thrombosis in veins but also in arteries if there is any atherosclerosis (pages 80–1). Researchers have now been studying women taking different brands containing the same oestrogen dose, but with varying doses of the same *progestogen*. An increasing number of conditions are found to become more frequent as the dose of progestogen increases, suggesting that the progestogen is important in causing the problem. A good example is blood pressure: the rate of diagnosis of high blood pressure (hypertension) was greatest in the pill with the highest dose of progestogen, least in the one with the lowest dose, as shown in Table 6. The dose of ethinyloestradiol is the same in all three pills (50 mcg).

Research reported in the early 1980s suggests that arterial diseases, especially heart attacks and strokes, are related in a similar way to increasing progestogen dose. Other examples of this are gallstones, acne, and thrombosis in superficial veins of the leg. It also appears that progestogen has important effects on body chemistry. This includes a *lowering* of one component of the blood lipids, high-density lipoprotein-cholesterol (HDL-cholesterol). Many experts think this substance is protective, so to reduce it may increase the risk of diseases of the circulation. Once again, the more progestogen is given, the greater the effect.

Blood glucose and insulin levels (especially the latter) tend also to be raised by a high content of progestogen. These changes imitate mild diabetes which is linked with an increased risk of atherosclerosis (page 81) – not that we can be sure this would be true when caused in a different way by the pill. But it is a further reason for concern to reduce the progestogenic strength of the formulations used.

Good effects may also depend on the progestogen. The reduction in the rate of benign breast disease mentioned on page 114, and the protective effect against symptoms, chiefly bleeding, from fibroids (page 104) are both greater the greater the progestogen content of the pill being given. Progestogen also appears to be linked with the reduced risk of pelvic infection

* **Table 6** Blood pressure according to dose of progestogen (RCGP Study)

Dose (milligrams) of progestogen (norethisterone acetate)	Rate of diagnosis of high blood pressure
4	13.9 per 1,000 women per year
3	12.3 ,,
1	8.2 ,,

(pages 103–4) and of cancer of the endometrium (page 122).

It seems clear that both progestogen and oestrogen can cause unwanted effects. For least effect on body chemistry, and probably also for lowest health risk, the minimum of both hormones should be used. This is how to give effect to that working rule we highlighted on page 74.

Progestogen-only pills (POPs) which are considered in Chapter 8, not only have no oestrogen, but also have less progestogen than most combined pills. So they ought by rights to have the lowest health risk of all, though too little research has yet been done to be quite sure about this (see pages 191, 195).

As might perhaps be expected, things are not that simple. As lower and lower doses were tried following the above reasoning, so there were more complaints about irregular bleeding from the women taking the modern pills. The failure rate also went up, much less obviously. All these problems were (are) naturally most frequent with POPs, although many women are well suited.

The new *variable-dose, so-called phased pills* seem to go some way to dealing with this dilemma. They reduce the progestogen as well as the oestrogen to the minimum available in combined pills, yet at the same time give most women an acceptable pattern of bleeding and are extremely effective at preventing pregnancy. So they are being more widely used (pages 168–71).

To sum up, the best advice for most pill-users in our present state of knowledge is to request a pill brand from among those giving the lowest available dose of both hormones. This policy not only reduces the risk of arterial and venous diseases in older women and possibly breast cancer in young women (see page 120); it also lessens the frequency of those so-called 'minor' side-effects listed on page 60. Higher doses should be reserved for the one exception: problems with bleeding (see pages 176–7).

6

The pill in perspective

Table 7 is a summary of most of the effects for which there is at least some evidence of a link with the pill. It is, of necessity, not entirely comprehensive. The emphasis to be given to any one effect depends on the answers to four important questions:

1. *How strong is the evidence?* Has it been consistently shown by more than one group of researchers? And/or is there a reason for expecting the effect such as a known change in body chemistry?

2. *How important is the condition being caused, worsened, or improved?*

3. *How large is the effect of the pill? (How many times more or less common is the condition in pill-users?)*

4. *How common is the condition anyway?*

Questions 3 and 4 are linked in the way to be described on page 141 (attributable risk), and they all apply to the good as well as the bad effects, of course. At the end of the day the conclusion, based on the answer to all four, depends on the individual judgement of the informed person, whether doctor or pill-user. Try answering these questions: which is the more important in deciding about the pill today, some very preliminary and unconfirmed evidence that the pill might increase the chance of a severe allergy in a tiny number of women? Or the certainty that abnormal pigmentation (chloasma) will develop in a larger number? And how do you match either with the certainty that an even larger number of pill-users will not get the iron deficiency anaemia due to heavy periods which they would otherwise suffer?

Although the actual amount of the extra risk or benefit may be hotly debated, the evidence linking them with the pill to some extent is at least adequate for the majority of the conditions mentioned in the last two chapters. In Table 7 those side-effects about which the evidence is weakest, or where the *net* effect of the pill is uncertain, are in brackets. There is no doubt that some women report loss of libido on the pill, for instance, but others report improvement: so loss of libido is in brackets because it is difficult to be sure what the *net* (overall) effect would be in a large group of pill-users.

You will notice that there is quite a long list of 'plus' points about the pill. You may have wondered in fact why two of them, the probable protective effects of the pill against cancer of the ovary and endometrium, have been omitted, along with some possible bad effects on cancer. As explained on pages 119–24, the reason is that the balance sheet for any link there may be (either way) between the pill and cancer cannot yet be drawn.

Figure 14 shows somewhat more clearly, because the facts are known from the RCGP Study, how frequent certain of the good and bad effects are, and by how much the pill increases or reduces their rate of occurrence.

If you have read right through the last two chapters, you are now perhaps overwhelmed by the number and variety of non-contraceptive effects of the pill. You may well be wondering why anyone can bring herself to use it. But suppose that you had instead been reading a very comprehensive account by a Casualty Surgeon of all the injuries and long-term complications which have been linked with road accidents – would you not similarly be wondering why people ever go anywhere by car? Yet all the different injuries due to cars added together are still uncommon enough to make it worth while for most people to use cars. Similarly, all the serious injuries which have been linked with the pill added together are uncommon. Indeed it would be a safe bet that most readers of this book will not know personally any family affected by a tragedy linked with the pill – whereas they probably know more than one resulting from road accidents. In spite of years of involvement with family planning, I am not aware of a case of a heart attack or stroke or any other serious unwanted effect occurring in any woman to whom I had personally prescribed the pill (though I have been asked to look after one or two who were prescribed the pill elsewhere, after such an event).

Table 7 Side-effects of the combined pill

Good Effects		Bad Effects	
Common	Uncommon or rare	Common	Uncommon or rare
• Acne – less with some pills	• (Duodenal ulcers – less)	• Absent bleeding in pill-free week	• Breast pain
• Benign breast disease – less	• Ectopic pregnancies – much less	• (Allergies)	• Chloasma or other skin troubles
• Breast tenderness – usually less	• (Endometriosis – less)	• Bleeding on pill-taking days	• Contact lens troubles
• Effective – nearly 100 per cent (hence relief of *fear of pregnancy*)	• Fibroids – fewer bleeding troubles	• Breast enlargement*	• Delayed return of fertility
• Good social effects (pages 15–16)	• Ovarian cysts – less	• Cramps and pains in legs, or in arms	• Eye troubles
• Intercourse – unaffected by the method	• Rheumatoid arthritis – less	• Cystitis and other urinary infections	• Fibroids – enlargement and sometimes pain
	• (Thyroid disease – less)	• (Depression)	• Gallstones
	• (Toxic shock – less)	• Erosion of cervix with increased vaginal discharge	• Heart attacks
			• Hypertension
			• Jaundice

Menstrual cycle improved:
- More regular bleeding
- Timing of 'periods' can be controlled (page 43)
- No ovulation pain
- Less pre-menstrual tension
- Less period pain
- Less heavy bleeding therefore
- Less anaemia

- Pelvic infection – less
- Poisoning – almost impossible
- Reversible – nearly 100 per cent
- (Trichomonas vaginitis – less)
- Unwanted hair growth – less with some pills
- Wax in the ears – less with some pills

- Fluid retention/bloatedness
- Gum inflammation
- Headaches
- (Loss of libido)
- Migraine
- Nausea
- Reduced resistance to some infections
- Unwanted social side-effects (pages 19–23).
- Weight gain*

- Milky fluid from breasts
- Phlebitis (thrombosis of superficial veins)
- Strokes
- Venous thrombosis with or without pulmonary embolism

Notes:
1. The order is alphabetical in each list. The various effects obviously differ enormously in their relative importance.
2. Brackets round an item mean that doubt remains about whether, or to what extent, the pill causes the effect.
3. Possible effects (either way) on cancers are omitted – see text.
4. *These may seem good effects to some underweight women.

137

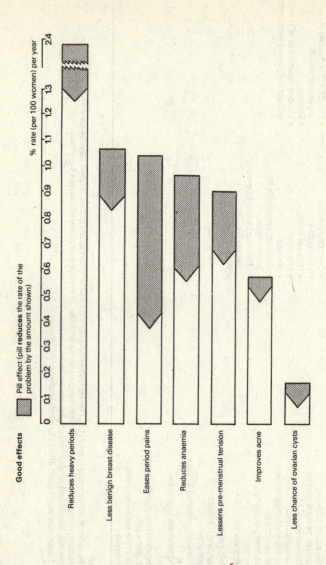

Good effects

Pill effect (pill **reduces** the rate of the problem by the amount shown)

% rate (per 100 women) per year

Reduces heavy periods

Less benign breast disease

Eases period pains

Reduces anaemia

Lessens pre-menstrual tension

Improves acne

Less chance of ovarian cysts

0 0.1 0.2 0.3 0.4 0.5 0.6 0.7 0.8 0.9 1.0 1.1 1.2 1.3 2.4

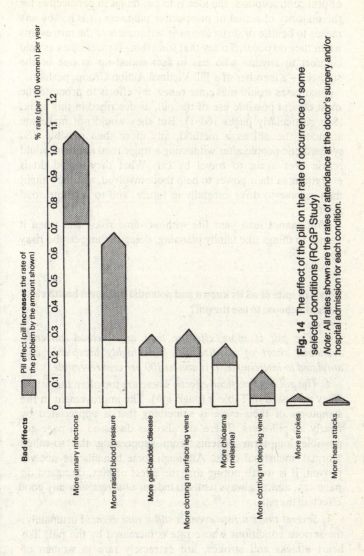

Fig. 14 The effect of the pill on the rate of occurrence of some selected conditions (RCGP Study)

Note: All rates shown are the rates of attendance at the doctor's surgery and/or hospital admission for each condition.

Bad effects

☐ Pill effect (pill **increases** the rate of the problem by the amount shown)

% rate (per 100 women) per year

- More urinary infections
- More raised blood pressure
- More gall-bladder disease
- More clotting in surface leg veins
- More chloasma (melasma)
- More clotting in deep leg veins
- More strokes
- More heart attacks

By emphasizing the rarity of all the dangerous complications of oral contraception, the idea is to put things in perspective for the majority of actual or prospective pill-users. It is not by any means to belittle or shrug away the seriousness of the rare events when they do occur. To say that something is rare comes as cold comfort to anyone who has in fact ended up as one of the statistics – a member of a Pill Victims' Action Group, perhaps.

Such cases would make me renew my efforts to promote the most careful possible use of the pill, as described in this book. (See particularly pages 160–1). But they would not make me abandon the pill as a method, any more than sensible and sympathetic people after witnessing a tragic road accident would refuse ever again to travel by car. What they would do is everything in their power to help those involved, and they might then resolve to drive carefully in future, and to promote road safety.

You cannot lead your life without some risks, and when it comes to things like family planning, doing nothing can be risky too.

Why – in spite of all its known and potential unknown health risks – might I choose to use the pill?

1. *The pill is more effective than any method currently available, short of sterilization. It is highly acceptable and unrelated to intercourse. It is almost 100 per cent reversible.*

2. *The pill has beneficial effects.* These are too often forgotten. They are listed in Table 7 (page 136). The improvement in the symptoms of their cycle is something that is appreciated by nearly all pill-users. There are also, as discussed on page 40, possible long-term benefits from suppressing the so-called 'normal' menstrual cycle. Although some benefits are not yet proven, it is worth noting that the effect of bias, discussed on page 125, almost always tends to hide or *underestimate* any good effects of the pill.

3. *Several times a rare event is still a rare event.* Fortunately, the serious conditions whose rate is increased by the pill, like heart attacks and strokes, are extremely rare in women of child-bearing years. So even if their rate is increased, that still

makes them very rare events. Suppose the pill increases the rate by a factor of 10. If the annual rate in non-users were one in 100,000, this would mean 10 cases in pill-users. But if the non-user rate were 10 in 100,000, there would be 100 cases per year in pill-users. The same relative risk factor of 10 means 90 extra cases in the second example but only 9 extra cases in the first. The extra cases are the so-called *attributable* or *excess* risk, and better convey the real importance of the pill effect. It is because the excess risk is so low for young ages (especially in non-smokers) that the relative risks, in the range of 2–6 for the various circulatory diseases, can be accepted. (The overall increased rate is about fourfold, see page 88.) Even for smokers, for example, the excess risk for those under 35 is only 10 per 100,000, whereas over the age of 45 it rises to 179 per 100,000 per year.

A small extra point which is perhaps worth mentioning is that all the research that has been done on the pill has failed to show up any condition which is new to science. It was always possible that the artificial hormones of the pill might cause some completely new disease. In fact, however, all the problems that are blamed on the pill happen also to women who have never had an artificial hormone in their lives, and as far as diseases of the circulation are concerned – which are far and away the most serious alleged risks – to men too. The average man is up to three times more at risk of circulatory disease, just because of his sex, than the average woman before her menopause. So if your partner of the same age is not scared about just being a man, perhaps you (especially if free of risk factors) can be relaxed about being a pill-using woman!

4. RISK ESTIMATES ARE AVERAGES, AND DO NOT NECESSARILY APPLY TO SUB-GROUPS. I put this point in capitals because it is so important. To understand it, please look back to page 82 and see how there, in the discussion on heart disease, I showed how the various estimated risks multiplied with each other and with the pill. But the opposite is also true: anyone without risk factors must have a much lower risk than average.

Perhaps an analogy may help to make this clearer. Insurance companies always require a high premium from students when they try to insure their cars; yet some of those students are very much safer drivers than the average (and may prove the fact in due course by having no accidents at all in the next twenty years). They always were safer drivers, but the risk estimates by the insurers had to be based on all kinds of students, including those who are irresponsible, who drive under the influence of alcohol, and so on. *To some extent – not altogether – those for whom pill-use is especially risky can now be identified.* The next chapter is partly about how this can be done. One way of putting it is: 'The pill is reasonably safe, but some women are dangerous.' As a result of better prescribing, the more 'dangerous' women should not now be using the method: and the *pill probably always was a lot less risky for the remainder (the safer women) than the overall estimates would suggest.*

5. *The risk estimates were based on research on higher-dose pills than are now in general use.* Pills which are low in dose of both oestrogen and progestogen have not yet been studied so thoroughly, and should be even safer (pages 131–3).

However, even following all the known guidelines for increasing the safety of pill-prescribing, including careful aftercare with blood pressure checks, trouble can still strike out of a clear blue sky. Risks can be lowered, but they can never be entirely eliminated.

6. *Pregnancy is fairly risky: the pill is very effective against pregnancy: so the risks of the pill may not be so worrying when the avoidance of pregnancy is taken into consideration.* In the past, this point has sometimes been made too strongly, and various graphs and diagrams produced which suggest that non-use of the pill is more dangerous than it is. But the main point still stands, and that is that when considering methods which are not so reliable against pregnancy as the pill, we have to add together two things: (i) the risk (if any) of the method itself and (ii) the risk of the pregnancies which will occur in a proportion of women due to failure of that method. No guarantee of safety can be given to any sexually active woman, whatever method of family planning she uses, or if she uses no method at all and keeps becoming pregnant. Pregnancy itself, whether its outcome is a baby or abortion or a miscarriage, still carries some risks even in countries like Britain or America, and far more in many less developed countries. One way or another (and most inequitably), for women sex is dangerous.

In fact, in the real-life situations of the RCGP, Oxford/FPA, and Walnut Creek Studies the death rate due to pregnancy in the non-pill-users was extremely small. This shows that on average the women concerned, or their partners, were reasonably careful using alternative methods of family planning and they had good medical care during their pregnancies. Neither of these facts is necessarily true for other women whose circumstances or behaviour are different. The sheath, for example, can have absolutely no health risk due to the method, and used consistently its effectiveness can be as good as that of the IUD. Nevertheless, everyone knows that unplanned pregnancies are more frequent among users of that method, partly because the rubber of which it is made may fail, but much more commonly because it is not used properly or regularly. The main conclusion is that *the risk of death, whether from the method or from pregnancy if the method fails, of all the recommended methods of birth control is low, and below the risk of child-bearing* if no method is used: except for older pill-users, particularly if they smoke. This is even more true wherever medical care for pregnant women is poor, and wherever, as tragically happens in many countries, dangerous illegal or back-street abortion is widely practised. Even in countries like Britain, young women are probably exposed to less danger, particularly if they do not smoke, in any given year if they take the pill than they would be if they were to have a baby.

Yet few who want a baby are put off by these known medical risks – nor should they be. So if you are young and free of risk factors your decision about the pill can be based more on other points, such as the convenience of the pill and the fact that it almost eliminates the fear of an unwanted pregnancy.

7. *Even the highest estimates of risk due to the pill are of the same order as many other risks many of us take every day.* Most of us are extremely vague and uninformed about the relative risks of daily activities. Smoking is a good example: accepted as 'normal' yet truly lethal (page 89). Many people accept comparable or greater dangers from those of the pill in their occupations, spare-time activities, or hobbies. Going for a drive in the car is an obvious example: on present estimates, if you are a young non-smoker, you are no more – indeed probably much less – likely to be seriously injured by being on the pill than on the roads. Going for a boating holiday on the River Thames is

143

less obviously risky – yet between 1973 and 1977, 55 people drowned on this one river alone, upstream from Teddington Lock. Some drowned while amusing themselves, some in attempting rescues, one after jumping from a bridge for a bet! Can you think of anything you could do which is completely safe? How about eating? In the USA approximately 3,000 people die each year from accidentally inhaling food, usually a piece of steak . . . One would think that keeping household pets is a safe enough hobby – yet the Brompton Hospital in London has recorded at least three deaths from allergy to hamsters. See Figure 1 for some more examples (page 6).

And what about unknown risks? If you stop to think about it, which most of us do not, there are many chemicals to which we are exposed every day which have never been studied as intensively as the pill. To take a simple example, how do we know that drinking coffee is an entirely safe habit? Until someone does something like the RCGP Study of the pill, which would mean taking 23,000 regular coffee-drinkers, and 23,000 comparable people who never touch the stuff, and then following up all 46,000 for ten years, keeping records of every death or attack of illness in the two groups, we shall never really know. There are other unknown risks which could be a lot higher: for instance, those due to pollution. Tens of thousands of powerful chemicals are released by industry into our environment, into the water we drink and the air we breathe, and also into our food. The dose of each may be small, but *nobody knows* just how much or little effect they could have on our health, either alone or in combination. There are other chemicals to which people expose themselves voluntarily: for instance, some hair dyes have been suspected of very rarely causing cancer. Again though, no one knows how rarely. And how about the chemicals that are added to much of the food we buy? These are sometimes thought to be essential as preservatives but often they are just for colouring, such as one called Brown FK which is used solely to make kippers and ginger-nut biscuits nice and brown. Here is something which could increase the rate of all kinds of diseases, and could be at least as dangerous – or as safe – as the pill. The point is we just do not know. *Taking risks is quite simply part of life*: or as the car-sticker puts it, 'Living is hazardous to your health.'

Please do not get me wrong: I am not arguing that two wrongs make a right, or rather that hundreds of wrongs make a right. Obviously there is no room for complacency about the risks of the pill. They should be reduced to the absolute minimum in the way that is described in the next chapter – and in the long run we hope the pill will be phased out and replaced by an entirely risk-free method (see Chapter 9). But right now the risks of the pill compare well with the known, let alone the unknown, risks to which we are all inevitably exposed. After considering its advantages and convenience, given the methods now available, the balance sheet of risks and benefits comes out favourable to the pill for many women.

The effect of the mass media on people's thinking about the pill

The strange thing is that often even with known serious risks, like smoking cigarettes, so many people are quite illogically not at all bothered: and yet they are terrified by other dangers (such as those of the pill in the absence of known risk factors) which are definitely not as great. Unbalanced press and TV publicity is often to blame. When did you last see a major article in a popular newspaper itemizing the risks of cigarettes, including interviews with the sufferers from smoking-related diseases like cancer of the lung, or with their relatives? Yet there have been numerous such articles about the pill, which quite fail to put its risks in perspective, in comparison to the risks of life generally, and especially the risks and problems of unwanted pregnancy. They also do not point out that sub-groups of pill-users, such as healthy young non-smokers, take even less than the average estimated risk.

It is well known that good news is not 'news'. For example, one of the good effects of the pill is the definite reduction in the chance of getting benign breast disease (see page 114). When this was first convincingly shown, the British Family Planning Association had just three press enquiries. By contrast the FPA switchboards were jammed in December 1969. This was the month when the Committee on the Safety of Medicines published a report showing that the (already small) risk to users of the pill of thrombosis in the deep veins of the leg could be

145

reduced still further if they were to switch to using lower-dose brands. Treatment of the story by some newspapers was so alarmist that a large proportion of users all over the world were frightened into stopping the pill altogether, often half-way through a packet and without taking alternative precautions. In Britain alone it is estimated that about 20,000 babies were born as a result, not to mention the pregnancies which were terminated (abortions). Similarly there was a clear rise in birth rate after the 1977 'pill scare'. That was when it was first announced that smoking and age were linked with the pill in causing an increased risk of arterial disease (pages 80–6). Partly because of this unbalanced reporting, many of those who gave up the pill – in 1969, again in 1977, and more recently – were the 'wrong' people. In other words, they were young; or older, but healthy and thin, active, non-smoking women. The pill could have been a godsend if their confidence in it had not been shattered. Presented later with a more complete picture of the risks and other problems of the alternatives to pill-use – or sometimes learning the hard way by having to have an abortion – some of these women made the voluntary and informed choice to go back on the combined pill.

Let me make four final points. First, *coincidences do happen*. Becoming ill sometimes is part of being human. Some people are inclined to blame on the pill every illness or symptom which occurs, in a past or present user. They need reminding of the logical implication of that, which is that no one who has never taken the pill would ever get ill at all!

Secondly, the risk of death or serious illness; though perhaps the major concern, it is certainly not the *only* factor to be considered when deciding between methods of family planning. As just one example, it has been shown by several experts that one of the very safest ways of birth control from the point of view just of avoiding death is to use a simple method of family planning like a spermicide – not usually recommended for use alone – and then, whenever a pregnancy occurs, to have a legal abortion. The facts are quite correct: there is no death rate using the simple method, and the death rate from the several abortions that would be necessary if this policy were followed would also be very low. Many readers of this book may be disturbed if not horrified by this suggestion; others might feel less strongly but

146

would agree that this is simply not the right way to go about things. Abortion is not family planning, though it is a fact that the difference between the two is becoming increasingly difficult to define (see page 206). Many, perhaps most, women would feel very uneasy if this approach were seriously recommended to them. That is not to say that some would not feel that an abortion was right in certain particular circumstances: it is the planning to have abortions regularly that would seem so wrong to many. I use this example chiefly to show that in the real world risks are not necessarily the most important factors which people consider when deciding what they themselves are going to do.

Thirdly, if one day a new contraceptive medicine which affects the whole system like the pill is devised, it will be worth considering the saying 'better the devil you know than the devil you don't'. In other words, we now know a lot about the pill which will inevitably take a long time to emerge during use of a new drug. It may perhaps be said of such a new drug that it is believed to have no unwanted effects on the circulation. That could be true, but then it might eventually prove to have more serious effects elsewhere in the body. 'Newer' is not necessarily 'better'.

Finally, in spite of what I have just said, as we saw earlier there are still many gaps in our knowledge about the pill. There are two ways of reacting to absent facts about the use of any drug, or of the pill. One person may say, *'there is not enough evidence of safety'*, another may say, *'there is no evidence of danger'*. A good example of what I mean can be found on page 196 of this book. A microscopic amount of progestogen gets into the breast milk if a woman is on the progestogen-only pill while breast-feeding. There is so far nothing to suggest that this could harm the baby in any way: but, of course, it might. I myself would say, 'there is no evidence that this harms the baby' and therefore I do prescribe this kind of pill at the request of a breast-feeding mother, after discussing the arguments with her. But other doctors can and do say, 'there is not enough evidence that this is entirely harmless to the baby': and this is an equally true statement, just the other way round. It is a bit like the difference between saying that a bottle is 'half full' and 'half empty'.

The point is that we are all having to decide on the basis of the

147

same present and absent facts. At the end of the day, it is a question of judgement. There are bound to be honest differences of opinion about how pills should be used – at least until the facts become absolutely unarguable, which is a rare event in the whole of medicine.

7

Who for the pill, and which pill for you?

Who should never take the pill?

We now know much better than before which women should never take the pill. If these are identified and advised to use other methods, then the remainder can use the pill with added confidence.

Whether the method is really to be forbidden in particular circumstances, or could perhaps be used with special care, is something about which experts frequently disagree. I think, however, that most doctors would say that another method should be used if anyone comes into one of the following ten categories. Doctors often call these *absolute contra-indications*.

1. *Past or present serious disease affecting the circulation*

(a) *Past history of any form of thrombosis* in any artery or vein anywhere in the body (see Chapter 4). The pill should be avoided whether the clotting occurred while previously taking the pill, whether in a situation which makes clotting more likely such as pregnancy or being confined to bed after an operation, or completely unexpectedly. All these troubles are rare, but the least uncommon would be clotting in one of the leg veins (pages 78–80).

(b) *Any past history of brain trouble diagnosed as a stroke* (page 83), whether thought to be due to blood clotting or to bleeding in the brain.

(c) *Extremely severe,* so-called 'crescendo' *migraine;* any migraine bad enough to be *treated with an ergotamine-containing drug* (pages 59, 97); or migraine of the *focal type.* Focal migraine shows itself by short-lived attacks of strange and very worrying symptoms (see page 85). There is a risk that these could lead to

149

an actual stroke in a woman on the pill. So any woman with migraine of this most unusual kind should either never go on the pill, or discontinue if she is already on it when the attack happens.

The same applies if such symptoms were ever to occur without a headache at all – this is thought to happen if there is a temporary interruption to the blood supply (ischaemia) of the brain; such attacks are therefore labelled *transient ischaemic attacks.*

(d) *An illness or condition which makes thrombosis more likely e.g. 'large dose' of a risk factor for disease of the circulation* (see page 81). What matters is how bad the risk factor is, and again, I think, most experts would agree that the following should avoid the pill:

- A woman who has *the problem of high or abnormal blood fats.* She is likely to know all about this, which is a condition that often runs in families; she will therefore be on a special diet and possibly drug treatment for it already. (See pages 74–5 and 81.)
- A woman with *severe diabetes, who already has signs of damage to the arteries or kidneys or changes affecting the eye.*
- *High blood pressure,* even when not on the pill. If there is a past history of blood pressure going up very significantly on the pill, and returning to normal when it was stopped, this also means that the combined pill should be avoided in future. Repeated readings at or above 160 mm for the systolic or 95 mm for the diastolic pressures – explained on page 87 – would in my view be too high both for starting and for continuing with the pill.
- *A very heavy cigarette smoker, such as a woman who smokes 50 or more cigarettes a day.*
- *A woman aged more than 45* (but see page 195).
- *A grossly obese woman* (say weighing over 50 per cent more than the correct weight for her height).

The above examples are where the single risk factor is strong enough on its own. More commonly, the decision to avoid the pill is based on:

- *Combinations of risk factors.* If two or more of the factors just mentioned apply, then the woman should avoid the pill completely, even though on their own they would not be bad enough for this to be recommended. For instance, any diabetic on treatment who is also a long-term smoker of 15 cigarettes or more should, in my view, avoid the method. You can easily work out other combinations which mean the same thing, by referring to the list on page 81.

- *Angina.* This means heart pain, of a type which is usually described as a constricting feeling around the chest, and perhaps going up the neck or down the arms, which is brought on by exercise. If this diagnosis has been given to such a pain, it means that the heart muscle is being temporarily supplied with too little blood. This happens because the coronary arteries are already affected by atherosclerosis, i.e. hardening of the arteries. So to reduce the chances of an actual coronary thrombosis, which would block the arteries altogether, the pill is certainly best avoided if any woman has been told she has angina.

* - *Some rareties.* This means other types of *heart disease,* including most varieties affecting the *heart valves; pulmonary hypertension* (high blood pressure in the circulation through the lungs); or a type of irregular heartbeat called *atrial fibrillation.*

There is a type of anaemia which affects only black people, called *sickle cell anaemia.* There are two forms of the condition and the milder one, which is pretty common, called sickle cell *trait*, does not contra-indicate the pill. But experts disagree about whether it must be avoided by women with the rarer sickle cell *anaemia.* They have attacks (so-called crises) from time to time, during which damaged red blood cells block up tiny arteries in the body. Theoretically these attacks might be worsened by oestrogen, promoting thrombosis and thus turning temporary blockages of the microcirculation into more permanent ones. Other evidence suggests that the progestogen of the pill might have favourable effects. Pregnancy is particularly dangerous in this condition, so some experts allow or even prefer a low-dose pill to be used – after full discussion. Other doctors would suggest either the POP (Chapter 8) or a quite different method. A particularly good choice might be Depo-Provera (page 202), if available. Research reported in 1982 showed this injectable contraceptive can be positively beneficial to women with sickle cell anaemia, by reducing the frequency of their painful crises.

The pill should be avoided altogether in those of the rare so-called *collagen diseases*, such as polyarteritis nodosa, and *blood diseases* – leukaemia, polycythaemia – in which there is already an increased likelihood of thrombosis.

The combined pill should normally be avoided or stopped in two more circumstances in which the risk of thrombosis is increased – particularly in veins of the legs (pages 78–9):

- *Long-term immobilization in bed.* Disabled women who are confined to a wheelchair *may*, however, be permitted to take an ultra-low-dose combined pill provided they are not overweight, and with special medical supervision.
- *For six weeks before and four weeks after any planned major operation.* Emergency operations can of course still be done, but it is most important to inform the doctor on your admission that you are taking the pill. Sterilization by laparoscopy (page 207) does not count as a major operation, so the combined pill need not be stopped beforehand.

As the progestogen-only pill does not affect clotting factors (page 191), most doctors agree that it can be continued up to and after major as well as minor operations.

2. *Present disease of the liver – whether or not connected with the pill*

If you are still suffering from the effects of damage to your liver after any kind of liver illness such as jaundice (commonly caused by *infectious hepatitis*), then the pill should be avoided – and, like alcohol, normally for six months after the relevant blood tests have become normal. Further tests of liver function may be advised after a month or so of pill-taking.

- The type of *jaundice of pregnancy* described on page 100 is so likely to recur on the pill that it would be sensible to avoid it.
- The disease *cirrhosis* of the liver, rare conditions of the liver and skin known as the *porphyrias*, and a couple of

exotic disorders affecting the excretion of bile, e.g. *Rotor syndrome, all contra-indicate the pill.*

* A history of one of the very rare *tumours of the liver* (page 124) means another method for the future.

* Finally, *gallstones* treated medically in the past could recur within the bile duct system, so it would normally be best to avoid the pill for the future. See page 101. If treated by removal of the gall-bladder take the advice of your surgeon.

3. Present disorder of the pituitary gland

This is a rare reason for not going on the pill, and the woman concerned should already be seeing a specialist. A woman with this problem may be told she needs no contraception. But if it is due to high blood levels of the hormone prolactin, pregnancy is not impossible; present advice is to avoid the pill, or use it only under the supervision of a specialist. (See page 113.)

4. Past history of actual cancer of any type which might be aggravated by the hormones of the pill

The reason is that the hormones of the pill *might* make the cancer more difficult to cure. The rule particularly applies to those very few women of child-bearing years who have had cancer of the breast or the ovary. The treatment of cancer of the cervix or lining of the uterus involves removing it (hysterectomy), so there is then no need to use the pill for family planning. Otherwise it is best if any woman who has had cancer of any type takes the advice of the specialist looking after her, and avoids the pill until she is given the 'all clear'.

Opinions vary about whether you should avoid the pill while being investigated for an abnormality in a cervical smear test, or subsequent to successful treatment by a cone biopsy (removal of the affected skin under anaesthetic), or the equivalent. The research discussed on page 122 is difficult to interpret. At the time of writing (1984), all experts are agreed that *attending without fail for the follow-up smears as instructed* (usually annually in this context) is the first priority. This gives such safe monitoring of the situation that if a woman really wants to continue taking the pill, she may do so; or if after full discussion she feels happier to use another method, this too is up to her.

153

5. *Recent abnormal bleeding, other than at period times, from the uterus: until its cause has been found*

The reason for avoiding the pill here is that any vaginal bleeding which is not clearly connected with periods – especially if it happens after intercourse – must be diagnosed as quickly as possible. This is to rule out disease of the uterus, commonly non-malignant growths called polyps, but very, very rarely cancer. As irregular bleeding of the type known as 'break-through' bleeding can occur on the pill, if this rule were not followed there is a risk that the diagnosis would be delayed, because the bleeding might be thought to be a side-effect of the pill. However, once the gynaecologist has definitely ruled out a serious cause for the abnormal bleeding, he will almost certainly then be happy for you to take the pill.

* 6. *Recent hydatidiform mole*

This was explained on page 123. Because of the risk of a rare cancer following it, oral contraception should be avoided until the special follow-up tests of hCG hormone levels are completely normal. After that, provided your gynaecologist agrees, the pill can be used in the normal way.

7. *Actual or possible pregnancy*

Here the reason for avoiding the pill until pregnancy has been ruled out is that there is an unproven risk, which if it exists must be very, very small, that pill-taking during pregnancy might damage the baby (see page 110).

8. *Past history of any serious condition occurring or worsening in a previous pregnancy, and known to be affected by sex hormones*

This is because, as I have said, the pill in some ways mimics pregnancy. *Jaundice of pregnancy* (page 100), the troublesome skin rash called *herpes gestationis* (page 117), and *chorea* (page 98) are three examples mentioned earlier. Deterioration of the inherited form of deafness called *otosclerosis* has been reported in pregnancy, but no increase in the number of patients with this trouble was shown among pill-takers in the RCGP Study.

9. *Important condition occurring on the pill in the past and considered to be due to it*

High blood pressure which definitely seems in a particular case

154

to be related to taking the pill has already been mentioned above; another example would be bad migraine occurring on the pill in a woman who never used to have the problem. This category also includes other conditions which can be found in Chapter 5, if your doctor feels that the pill is very likely to blame: for example, the severe skin rash erythema multiforme, which may be due to an allergy to one of the hormones contained in the pill.

10. *Unconvinced that the pill is right for you*

If you or your partner cannot feel confident about using the pill, after discussing things with your doctor, or reading a book like this, then obviously you should avoid it. A doctor may perhaps insist that there is no medical reason why you should not take it, but you should always have the final word.

Notice, by the way, that several of the above ten reasons for avoiding the pill are not necessarily permanent.

Who should be very cautious about taking the pill and then only with special medical supervision? (See page 160 for what is meant by 'special supervision')

This means women with *relative contra-indications:* risk factors which do not necessarily mean that the pill should be avoided altogether, but they do require careful consideration *relative* to the other risks – including those of pregnancy – that are faced by that woman, and the acceptability of alternatives to the pill.

For example, diabetes in a young woman increases the risk of disease of the circulation, as does the pill (page 81); but it also increases the risks of pregnancy and delivery above the average. So if no other acceptable method can be found the pill could still be a reasonable choice for short-term use after discussion and with careful medical supervision.

These relative contra-indications are mostly obvious after reading Chapters 4 and 5. The important ones are listed here: if more than one applies, particularly of the first seven below, then the pressure to move to another method rather than the pill increases.

1. *A family history of disease of the circulation*

This means a history of thrombosis – such as coronary thrombosis or deep-vein thrombosis in the legs – or of stroke, occurring in a near-relative *at a young age:* say under 45. Heart attacks in young member(s) of your family may mean artery trouble and your doctor may perhaps arrange for measurement of your blood fats (page 81). Should abnormal levels be found, then you will probably be told to avoid the pill altogether (see page 150). If not, and in cases where the family history is not so strong, it may be all right for you to go on the pill with medical supervision.

The doctor should also be told if there is a tendency in your family to raised blood pressure.

2. *Diabetes*

Diseases of the circulation are already more likely in diabetics, so in my view it is preferable to avoid any extra risk in the same direction. In practice, however, some young diabetics who are free of any signs of complications of the disease are on this method, because they need maximum protection against pregnancy. There may be no satisfactory alternative. If so they occasionally need to increase their insulin dose and they should naturally be seen at frequent intervals by a doctor. It is even more important for diabetics than it is for other people not to smoke. It would be important for them to be on the lowest possible dose of pill, perhaps a triphasic, pages 68–71, or even better the POP (page 194), and for as short a time as possible. They will probably be encouraged to have their babies as young as their circumstances allow. Then they will most likely be advised to transfer to another method or perhaps be sterilized as soon as they complete their family.

Women with a strong family history of diabetes, or who are overweight, or who had the very mild blood test changes of diabetes in pregnancy, or who gave birth to a baby weighing more than 4.5 kilograms, all need to be carefully observed on the pill. They usually should have the test mentioned on page 74 (the Glucose Tolerance Test) before and perhaps a couple of months after going on the combined pill.

3. *High blood pressure*

Like diabetes, this was also mentioned in the previous section. Everything really depends on how bad the blood pressure is, how young the woman is, whether there are any other risk factors present, and whether any alternative methods of family planning are acceptable. Readings *around* 140 systolic/90 diastolic (page 87) will normally indicate just frequent check-ups. Above those levels, your doctor may advise you to abandon the combined pill; and this would certainly be necessary if the values were above 160/95. You might then try the progestogen-only type (Chapter 8). It is important to remember that a rise in blood pressure may sometimes be a sign of another risk which is *coupled with it* (see page 86). So even a small rise can be important if there are other risk factors already – e.g. in a smoker.

A past history of raised blood pressure, perhaps in pregnancy, or of kidney disease, means that there should be more frequent checks of the blood pressure during use of the pill.

4. *Heavy cigarette-smoking*

Remember that this is defined as 15 or more cigarettes a day. It multiplies the increased risks of circulatory diseases three times or more: both when not taking the pill and when taking it. It really boils down to: 'you pays your money and you takes your choice', either your cigarettes or the pill! If you cannot stop smoking altogether, it will always do you good to cut down; and unless another risk factor appears such as your passing the age of 30 to 35, you are not someone who absolutely *must* avoid the pill.

But ideally no pill-user would ever smoke, at all.

5. *Age of more than 30 to 40* (see Table 4, page 90, and page 128)

Nothing suddenly happens on your fortieth birthday (or on your thirtieth birthday if you are a heavy smoker) which *suddenly* makes it risky to be on the pill. The risk increases steadily with age and all that your birthday means is that it is now time to reassess your family planning method, if you have not done so earlier.

If after reference to Table 4 and discussion with your doctor you decide you must stop the combined pill – all is not lost! This may be a very good time for you to transfer to the progestogen-only pill. Table 13 on pages 221–3 in the last chapter of this book may also help you to decide between the various possibilities.

6. *Long duration of use of the pill while still under 35 – say ten years or more*

There is a lot of uncertainty about this (see pages 126–30). So after 10 years it would be sensible to review your situation, with your doctor, and to *consider* transferring to another method. The suggested *maximum* duration is 20 years, reduced to 10–15 years if another of the headings 1–7 here applies to you as well.

7. *Excessive weight* (page 82). *Marked varicose veins* (page 80)

These were discussed earlier. Both tend to be associated with an increased risk of thrombosis, but probably indirectly. Both can also become more problematic in pill-takers. Overweight is of course something about which you can, in theory, do something yourself.

For women in all the above categories a pill which is particularly low in dose/potency of *progestogen* – as well as oestrogen – is preferable, as explained on page 132.

Now I come on to some reasons for extra caution which are not to do with diseases of the circulation.

8. *Scanty or very irregular periods or their absence (amenorrhoea)*

Following use of the pill, lack of egg-release and therefore periods for six months to a year or longer does occur in a very few women (see page 109). Some of these may require special treatment in order to achieve a pregnancy. The small number with this very treatable problem can be reduced by a *flexible* policy of preferring other methods for women whose periods are infrequent or absent, especially if the women are very underweight; or were older than usual at the time of their first-ever period. Another factor to consider would be the local availability of modern tests and treatments for amenorrhoea.

It is illogical for the combined pill to be used, as it has been in the past, in young women who do not require it for family planning simply to 'regularize' infrequent and irregular periods. After all, pill 'periods' are entirely artificial (see page 38). On the other hand, if *investigation* shows no reason (such as raised prolactin, page 153) to avoid it, one of the very lowest-dose pills from Figure 15, pages 165–7, may be used if desired. Much depends on other factors in an individual case such as the acceptability of alternative methods. What might they be? The best would be

158

barriers such as the sheath or the cap. The IUD would be a very poor choice in these circumstances as it is linked with a much less treatable cause of reduced fertility (see page 221). In teenagers, starting the pill should always be delayed until regular periods have become properly established (see page 115).

9. *Fluid retention*
Too much fluid in the body can be risky for a few people who have certain types of *heart and kidney disease*. The pill tends to cause retention of some fluid (page 76) so special care is needed if such women are to use it.

Some women who suffer from *migraine* (page 96), *epilepsy* (page 97), and *asthma* (page 99) are more prone to get attacks when taking the pill. Others notice an improvement. Various changes in body chemistry, including the fluid retention just mentioned, may be involved. The uncertainty means that women with any of these three conditions need special advice and supervision if they go on the pill – *especially in the matter of changes in the symptoms of migraine* (page 85).

10. *Severe depression* (see page 93)
A history of really bad depression which required treatment for a long time with drugs for 'nerves' means the pill should normally be avoided. However, there could be a few exceptions to the rule.

11. *The use of interfering drugs – especially treatments for tuberculosis and epilepsy.* See page 57, also 171–2.
Page 58 lists those drugs which may cause problems. The main practical points here are to make sure that the doctor who prescribes you the pill knows what, if any, other drugs you take; and if you are about to start any new treatment to remind the doctor that you are a pill-taker. If alternative methods do not suit you, it may be reasonable for you to continue taking the pill. However, unlike the other relative contra-indications in this list, this one means that it is best for you to use one of the 50 mcg pills from Table 9 (page 163) rather than the 'preferred' ultra-low-dose pills of Table 8. This is because of the need to overcome the effect of the interference by the other drug which may be causing the pill to be less effective. It is also very important for you to go back promptly to your clinic or family doctor if you ever get 'breakthrough' bleeding or fail to get a 'period' during the pill-free week.

The same rules apply to anyone who already has a disease which may interfere with absorption of the pill hormones, especially due to constant diarrhoea (see page 56). This can happen, for example, following operations for gross obesity.

* 12. *Should the pill be used by people who already have other chronic (long-term) diseases?*

It all depends. There is obviously no space to consider them all here, but if you look in the Index you will find that a number, such as diabetes, have already been discussed. Some women who have diseases which lead to very heavy periods, such as those on artificial kidney treatment – or who have difficulty because of disablement in coping with naturally rather heavy periods – positively benefit from the light ones that the pill gives. If women with the allergic and auto-immune disorders considered on page 118 go on the pill, the result is often unpredictable, so close medical supervision is essential. Hodgkin's disease, multiple sclerosis, myasthenia gravis and sarcoidosis are believed to be neither worsened nor improved by the pill. But more research is needed, into these and other diseases too numerous to mention. The main rules are:

(a) discuss the whole matter with your doctor, as usual balancing known and unknown risks of the pill *in your situation* against those of pregnancy and the pros and cons of alternative methods;
(b) be sure that you are *carefully followed up* by a doctor or specialist who knows the full story.

13. *Abnormal cervical smears under observation or treated.* See pages 122 and 153.

14. *Breast cancer in close relative(s) or other risk factor*

To play safe, while awaiting more research, short-term use is preferred – especially by teenagers. See pages 120–1, 129.

How then can use of the pill be made safer? An ideal scheme

- First of all, *women to whom something applies from the first list above* (pages 149–55) *should use some other method.*
- Secondly, *those with relative contra-indications* (pages 155–60) should *either avoid it or use it under special medical supervision.* This means being seen at a clinic or surgery more often than usual, being told if there is anything special to look out for so as to return earlier if

necessary, and sometimes having special tests done. It also means being ready to discontinue the pill should a condition worsen, or a new risk factor or problem appear – such as raised blood pressure.

- Thirdly, *all women, especially those with risk factors, should use pills with the lowest acceptable amount of both hormones* – often starting with the lowest of all (page 175) – *with duration of use being periodically reassessed* (page 129).

- Fourthly, *all pill-users should be seen regularly* by a trained person who can answer their questions, and check their weight and *especially their blood pressure* (page 130). Every pill-user should be encouraged to contact the trained person at short notice should a symptom arise – whether it is an annoying or irritating one, or a worrying one such as those in the list on page 61. Particularly important would be the first onset of *migraine headaches* while on the pill, or any change in related symptoms (page 85). Pill-users should also practise monthly *self-examination of the breasts* (page 121) and have regular *cervical smears* (page 122).

In summary, the SAFER women (see page 142) should use the modern SAFER pills, with careful MONITORING.

What pills are available?

Table 8 lists those pills containing less than 50 mcg of oestrogen which are currently available in Britain. This category includes the first-choice pills for all women. I say this first because they do provide enough hormones to be extremely effective against pregnancy. Provided they are taken regularly, they seem to be as effective for most women as the pills containing 50 mcg of oestrogen which are all shown in Table 9. However, the 'room-for-error' factor is probably less. So it is even more important that pills are not taken late or missed. Secondly, the main reason for choosing from these pills is that, as they give less total hormone dose, they should according to present knowledge give rise to less unwanted effects – both of the dangerous and 'nuisance' type. But the Table 8 pills are not all equivalent. There are some which give more progestogen than others and

* **Table 8** Ultra-low-dose combined pills with less than 50 micrograms of oestrogen available in Britain

162

Name of pill	Dose of oestrogen (ethinyloestradiol) in micrograms	Name and dose of progestogen in milligrams	Remarks
Group A		*levonorgestrel*	
Ovran 30	30	0.25	
Eugynon 30	30	0.25	
Ovranette	30	0.15	
Microgynon 30	30	0.15	
Trinordiol	30, 40, 30[32.4]	0.05, 0.075, 0.125[0.092]	Doses are for first 6 days, then 5 days, then 10 days respectively. Logynon ED has 7 'blank' tablets for the no-treatment days.
Logynon			
Logynon ED			
Group B		*desogestrel*	
Marvelon	30	0.15	
Group C		*norethisterone*	
Norinim	35, 35[35]	1.0	Doses are for first 7 days, then 14 days, respectively.
Neocon 1/35	35, 35[35]	0.5, 1.0[0.83]	
Binovum	35, 35[35]	0.5, 1.0[0.83]	
Trinovum	35, 35, 35[35]	0.5, 0.75, 1.0[0.75]	Doses are each given for 7 days.
Brevinor	35	0.5	
Ovysmen	35	0.5	
Group D		*norethisterone acetate*	
Loestrin 30	30	1.5	
Loestrin 20	20	1.0	
Group E		*ethynodiol diacetate*	
Conova 30	30	2.0	

Notes: 1. Each group uses a different progestogen. All are 21-day regimes. 2. The pills which are bracketed together have identical formulas, and the main difference is that they are marketed by different firms. 3. Within the body, all the progestogens in pills from Groups C to F are largely converted into norethisterone. Groups A and B are different, as discussed on page 164. 4. Average daily

Name of pill	Name and dose of progestogen in milligrams	Remarks
Group A Ovran Eugynon 50	*levonorgestrel* } 0.25	Eugynon 50 differs by also containing 0.25 mg of inactive progestogen hormone
Group C Norinyl-1 Norinyl-1/28 Ortho-Novin 1/50	*norethisterone* } 1.0	1. All 3 contain mestranol – as the oestrogen – this is very similar to ethinyloestradiol 2. Norinyl-1/28 includes 7 'blank' tablets for the 7 days off treatment
Group D Anovlar 21 Gynovlar 21 Norlestrin Orlest 21 Minovlar Minovlar ED	*norethisterone acetate* 4.0 3.0 2.5 } 1.0	Minovlar ED includes 7 blank tablets (like Norinyl-1/28)
Group E Ovulen 50	*ethynodiol diacetate* 1.0	
Group F Minilyn	*lynestrenol* 2.5	This is the only pill with 22 tablets to be taken followed by a 6-day break

See notes 1–3 of Table 8.

should therefore be avoided (page 132), unless there is a special reason (such as those discussed on page 178).

Tables 8 and 9, and Figure 15 – which is about to be explained – are based on those pills at present available in Britain. However, if you live elsewhere, you should still be able to follow the discussion in the rest of this chapter if you refer to the World Directory of pill names (page 266). This shows the individual formulations and the brand names used all over the world, including those equivalent to the ones in the Tables and Figures. Perhaps the simplest thing would be to use a ball-point pen to change the names here to those given to the brands used in your country.

Pill ladders

Please look at Figure 15: you will find it useful to keep referring to it throughout the rest of this chapter. The pills from both Tables 8 and 9 have been brought together in this figure, and those which contain the same progestogen in each of the Groups A to F have been arranged in ladders, also labelled A to F. They are ranked one above the other like the rungs of a ladder, in approximate order of total hormone dose being given to the body. The recommended pills are below the second horizontal line, and below them – 'at ground level' so to speak because so little hormone is being taken – are the progestogen-only pills.

The main message of Figure 15 is that, like all ladders, the lower down you are the less risk there is. For most women a pill below the *second* line in the figure is preferable. Although the brands in the middle section (Eugynon 30/Ovran 30 and Conova 30) are low in oestrogen, they have strong progestogen effects which are best avoided – see pages 131–3. But there can be special *medical* reasons for using them – see page 178.

Within any one ladder, the ranking order is clear, as you can see by checking the doses given in Tables 8 and 9. Between the ladders C, D, E and F it is also probably true that pills on the same rungs (say, Minilyn and Norlestrin) are more or less equivalent in their contraceptive dose (though *not* necessarily equivalent in their capacity to produce side-effects in an individual woman). The reason for this similarity is because all the four progestogens in pills from these ladders finish up, after various chemical reactions in the body, mainly as the one active hormone, norethisterone. Likewise the oestrogen mestranol in the two Norinyl-1 brands and in Ortho-Novin 1/50 ends up, after conversion in the body, mainly as the standard oestrogen of all the other pills, ethinyloestradiol.

Ladders A and B are different

That is why they are shown separately in Figure 15. The progestogens concerned called levonorgestrel (LNG) and desogestrel (DSG) are not transformed into norethisterone. They are both very 'potent', so small doses are required. Indeed, for minimal disturbance of the body's chemistry, *it is even more important than for the other ladders that a pill from a low rung in ladder A should normally be chosen.*

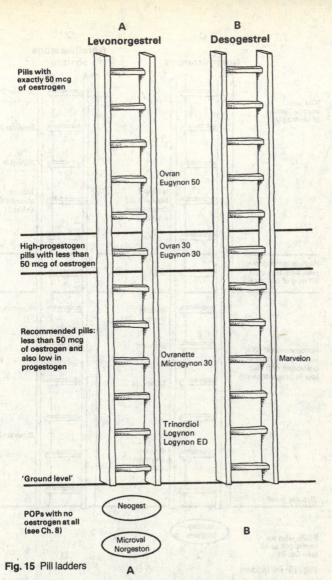

A
Levonorgestrel

B
Desogestrel

Pills with exactly 50 mcg of oestrogen

Ovran
Eugynon 50

High-progestogen pills with less than 50 mcg of oestrogen

Ovran 30
Eugynon 30

Recommended pills: less than 50 mcg of oestrogen and also low in progestogen

Ovranette
Microgynon 30

Marvelon

Trinordiol
Logynon
Logynon ED

'Ground level'

POPs with no oestrogen at all (see Ch. 8)

Neogest

Microval
Norgeston

B

A

Fig. 15 Pill ladders

Notes: 1. Within each ladder the same progestogen is used.   2. The rungs are ranked as far as possible according to the total hormone dose being given; lowest = least dose.   3. Refer to the World Directory of pill names (page 266) if living outside Britain.

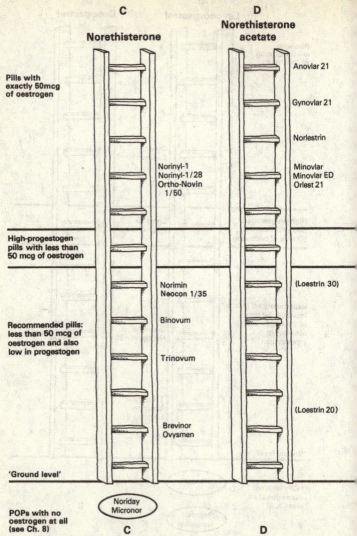

Fig. 15 Pill ladders

Notes: 1. Within each ladder the same progestogen is used. 2. The rungs are ranked as far as possible according to the total hormone dose being given: lowest = least dose. Loestrin 20 and 30 are difficult to classify: low/very low oestrogen dose but a medium to high dose of progestogen. 3. Refer to the World Directory of pill names (page 266) if living outside Britain.

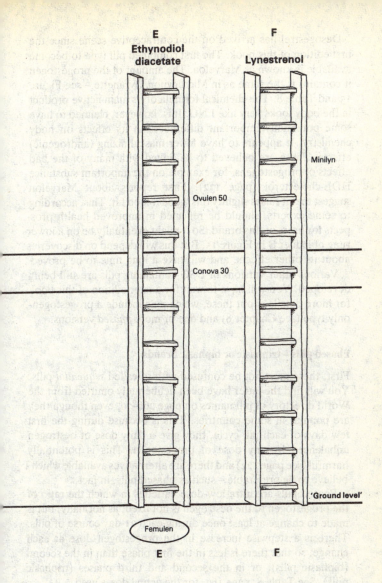

E
Ethynodiol diacetate

F
Lynestrenol

Minilyn

Ovulen 50

Conova 30

'Ground level'

Femulen

E   F

Desogestrel has arrived on the contraceptive scene since the first edition of this book. The first combined pill type to become available is known as Marvelon. The amount of the progestogen it contains is the same as in Microgynon/Ovranette – see Figure 15 and Table 8. The chemical formula of its main active product in the body looks very like LNG. It is, however, claimed to have some potentially important differences in its effects on body chemistry. It appears to have fewer masculinizing (androgenic) effects. These are believed to be linked with many of the bad effects of progestogens, for example on the important substance HDL-cholesterol (page 132). First reports about Marvelon suggest that it raises slightly this 'good' blood fat. This, according to some experts, should be reflected in improved health prospects for users of this brand. So it might eventually be on a lower rung of ladder B in Figure 15. But this will depend on discoveries about its other effects, and will take a long time to be proved.

Various other versions of DSG-containing pills are still being developed. You will have to wait for a later edition of this book for more details about these, which may include a progestogen-only type (see Chapter 8) and one or more *phased* versions.

Phased pills – triphasic or biphasic brands

First, these must not be confused with so-called *sequential* pills. You will find the latter have been deliberately omitted from the World directory of pill names on page 266–70, even though they are popular in some countries. This is because during the first few days of each pill cycle, they give a daily dose of oestrogen unbalanced by any dose of progestogen. This is potentially harmful (see page 122) and there are alternatives available which I believe to be preferable – such as phased pills, in fact.

Phased pills are ultra-low-dose varieties in which the ratio of the progestogen to the oestrogen is not fixed, as normally, but is made to change at least once during each 21-day course of pills. There is a stepwise increase in the progestogen dose at each change, so that there is less in the first phase than in the second (biphasic pills), or in the second and third phases (triphasic pills). See Table 8, page 162, for the actual doses used.

Although like all combined pills the phased types take away the menstrual cycle (page 38), the hormones are given in a way which does somewhat imitate the normal monthly variations. It is claimed that this is a good thing for general health. That will take many years to prove. But one thing is already clear: under the microscope a more normal-looking lining to the uterus does develop, and comes away better during each 'period' (withdrawal bleed). So although they give such a small and therefore probably safer dose of the pill hormones (page 133), they give a better bleeding pattern than similar fixed-dose versions would. For example, Trinordiol/Logynon is as good for this as the higher-dose brands Ovranette/Microgynon 30.

Studies of the body chemistry of users of biphasic and triphasic pills have tended to show reduced effects (sometimes no effects) on important substances such as HDL-cholesterol (page 132), as compared with fixed-dose brands. This is chiefly because the latter have to give a higher dose to control bleeding.

With phased pills treatment normally *starts* on the first day of a period, with no extra precautions necessary – unless it is the Every Day type (follow the rules of the package insert). Always take the phases of pills in the correct order, as shown by the arrows.

If transferring from another pill higher up a ladder, it is best to follow the rule on page 59 – i.e. immediate transfer from the last pill of the old packet to the first of the phased pill, again with no extra precautions. Take your doctor's advice if transferring to an Every Day variety. If you transfer on the particular day during the last week of the previous pill packet which allows you to take the first *active* hormone-containing pill without there being any break between packets, no extra pregnancy risk will result. In the case of Logynon ED this means *starting with the first (pink) Saturday tablet in the sequence, having stopped the previous brand whenever you reached the last Friday pill* – i.e. generally wasting the last few tablets in the previous packet. If, however, you follow the rules of the package insert, you will start on the first day of your withdrawal bleed after the previous packet. As this usually means taking some 'dummy' pills first, another method such as the sheath should then be used as well for the next fourteen days. The reason for these extra precautions is explained on page 59.

It will obviously be easier to understand the last paragraph if you have the relevant pill packets in front of you.

Now for a summary of the main pros and cons of these pills.

Advantages of phased pills

1. Little effect on most substances measured in the blood. But this is also true of some other ultra-low-dose brands giving a fixed dose (which may otherwise suit the woman).

2. *Almost* 100 per cent effective, like other pills, if taken regularly (but see below).

3. Good control of the bleeding pattern.

4. Logynon and Trinordiol are relatively oestrogen dominant (page 178) compared with the nearest equivalent in Figure 15. This can help symptoms such as *acne*.

5. Possibly: long-term benefits due to imitating the menstrual cycle(?).

Problems of phased pills

1. Reduced margin for error if women tend to forget pills.

2. Rather easier to get confused and hence to make pill-taking errors, as there are two or three phases of tablets to take in the right order. What is more, some versions do not have the day of the week against the tablet.

3. Explaining how to use them takes a bit more of the doctor's or nurse's time.

4. Some women complain of pre-menstrual symptoms during the final phase of tablet-taking, such as breast tenderness.

5. A very few women transferring from fixed-dose pills complain of a heavier or more painful flow during periods.

6. Phased pills are not a good choice if progestogen dominance required (especially to control benign breast disease – page 114).

7. Postponing periods is a little more difficult than with fixed-dose pills. Page 43 describes the usual way to do this, by taking two packets in a row. With a phased pill that might well not work; the switch from the higher progestogen dose of the last phase to the low dose of the first phase tends to cause withdrawal bleeding. So there are two alternatives:

(a) *Take extra pills from the last phase of a different packet.* This will give a maximum of ten days' postponement with Trinordiol/Logynon, for example, using the yellow tablets; or seven days using the third phase of Trinovum (which can be conveniently snapped off).

(b) *Interpose a packet of the next higher brand up the same ladder* in Figure 15. You should make an 'instant' switch from the phased pill to and from the fixed-dose brand – i.e. no days without pill-taking till the end of the whole nine-week sequence. This should give at least six weeks free of bleeding, perhaps longer. *Example:* After her last Binovum pill on, say, a Monday, Mrs Jones takes the first pill (marked Tuesday) from a Norimin packet. Three weeks later she takes the Tuesday pill from the first (white) section of another Binovum packet. She expects to see a small amount of bleeding in the next few days; but, whether she does see some bleeding or not, she carries on to the end of the Binovum packet before taking the usual seven-day break.

If in doubt discuss this with a doctor or nurse.

All in all it is not yet certain from body chemistry research or in practice, that it would be best for all women to transfer to phased pills. Yet they do form a useful addition to the available range.

Which pill should be chosen?

Even if you have been on one of the brands above half way on one of the ladders in Figure 15 for years with no problems, I would recommend discussing with your doctor whether it might not now be better to try taking a pill from a low rung on the same ladder. Obviously many people are reluctant to 'change a winning team' but, provided you follow the instructions on page 59, you will be quite safe from pregnancy during the change-over and later. You might also even notice that some mild symptoms you have lived with on the previous pill will now improve.

The only likely problem you may run into with an ultra-low-dose pill like this is a slightly irregular bleeding pattern. This is usually only for the first two or three months while your body is getting used to it.

Can there be good reasons for not being on a below-the-lines pill in Figure 15?

Yes: not every woman is suited by one of these ultra-low-dose pills. There is that reduced 'margin for error' which means that they may not be good for those who often forget to take tablets;

nor for those who have to take interfering drugs or who may have absorption problems. Poor absorption is relatively common among women in less developed countries (page 125). And some ordinary pill-users find difficulty in obtaining a good regular bleeding pattern with the lowest-dose brands. One containing more of either hormone may then be prescribed (see below).

As all these examples have in common the fact that the blood level of the pill hormones is likely to be a little reduced, from your body's point of view it is possible (though not certain in every case) that this is almost the same thing as being on one of the ultra-low-dose pills. The situation is roughly equivalent to climbing up a moving staircase which is going down.

Tailoring the pill to you

Doctors have in the past produced elaborate schemes from which they claimed to be able to choose the right pill for each woman's hormonal make-up. Unfortunately, they never really worked, chiefly because of too little information on the effects of different formulas; and also because of the variation between women, in the way their bodies absorb and react to the pill's hormones. For example, complaints like nausea, vomiting, breast discomfort, menstrual cramps, and delay in return of periods post-pill, all tend to be commoner in underweight women. (Though weight is not otherwise a useful guide as to how strong a pill to give.)

Regardless of weight, on comparing different women at a set time after taking the same brand of tablet very different blood levels have been found. Levels of the progestogens norethisterone and levonorgestrel can vary tenfold between women. Furthermore, relatively high levels of hormone (in this case the oestrogen) have been found in those pill-takers who developed high blood pressure. A likely conclusion is that many unwanted effects, both serious and 'minor', are connected with having unnecessarily high blood levels: caused either by unusually efficient absorption or inefficient elimination of the hormones.

Since it is impractical to measure blood levels routinely, and low levels do have the problem of causing irregular bleeding (page 133), doctors have tended in the past to give some women more hormone than might have been necessary. In the light of the new data here and elsewhere in this new edition, I am now

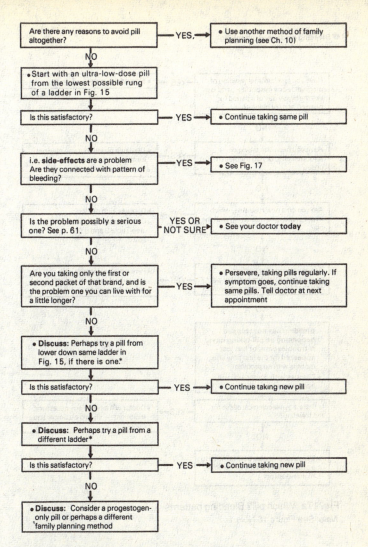

| Are there any reasons to avoid pill altogether? | — YES, → | • Use another method of family planning (see Ch. 10) |

NO ↓

• Start with an ultra-low-dose pill from the lowest possible rung of a ladder in Fig. 15

| Is this satisfactory? | — YES → | • Continue taking same pill |

NO ↓

| i.e. side-effects are a problem Are they connected with pattern of bleeding? | — YES → | • See Fig. 17 |

NO ↓

| Is the problem possibly a serious one? See p. 61. | YES OR NOT SURE → | • See your doctor today |

NO ↓

| Are you taking only the first or second packet of that brand, and is the problem one you can live with for a little longer? | — YES → | • Persevere, taking pills regularly. If symptom goes, continue taking same pills. Tell doctor at next appointment |

NO ↓

• Discuss: Perhaps try a pill from lower down same ladder in Fig. 15, if there is one.*

| Is this satisfactory? | — YES → | • Continue taking new pill |

NO ↓

• Discuss: Perhaps try a pill from a different ladder*

| Is this satisfactory? | — YES → | • Continue taking new pill |

NO ↓

• Discuss: Consider a progestogen-only pill or perhaps a different family planning method

Fig. 16 Which pill?

Notes: 1. 'Discuss' means *discuss at next visit with doctor or nurse: they will not take kindly to being told by you what to do next*. 2. If moving down a ladder, start the new packet without any break. 3.* At the points marked, choice of new pill is sometimes based on oestrogen or progestogen dominance (see page 178).

173

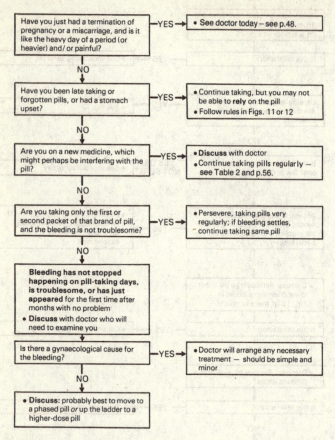

● **Bleeding on days of pill-taking**
(i.e. 'breakthrough' bleeding)

Have you just had a termination of pregnancy or a miscarriage, and is it like the heavy day of a period (or heavier) and/or painful?	—YES→ • See doctor today – see p.48.

NO ↓

Have you been late taking or forgotten pills, or had a stomach upset?	—YES→ • Continue taking, but you may not be able to **rely** on the pill • Follow rules in Figs. 11 or 12

NO ↓

Are you on a new medicine, which might perhaps be interfering with the pill?	—YES→ • **Discuss** with doctor • Continue taking pills regularly – see Table 2 and p.56.

NO ↓

Are you taking only the first or second packet of that brand of pill, and the bleeding is not troublesome?	—YES→ • Persevere, taking pills very regularly; if bleeding settles, continue taking same pill

NO ↓

Bleeding has not stopped happening on pill-taking days, is troublesome, or has just **appeared** for the first time after months with no problem
• **Discuss** with doctor who will need to examine you

↓

Is there a gynaecological cause for the bleeding?	—YES→ • Doctor will arrange any necessary treatment — should be simple and minor

NO ↓

• **Discuss**: probably best to move to a phased pill *or* up the ladder to a higher-dose pill

Fig. 17a Which pill? Bleeding patterns
Note: See Figure 16 Note 1.

recommending a new policy. In general, and with some exceptions, *all new prescriptions should be for a brand of pills from the lowest rung of one of the ladders* (but not normally Loestrin 20, as its oestrogen dose is too low for acceptable control of the bleeding cycle). This policy will avoid giving any woman

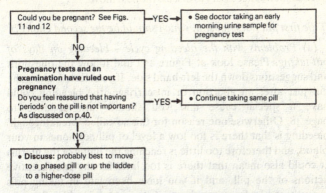

● **No bleeding at all during pill-free week** (no 'periods') – at least two missed*

| Could you be pregnant? See Figs. 11 and 12 | —YES→ | ● See doctor taking an early morning urine sample for pregnancy test |

NO

| Pregnancy tests and an examination have ruled out pregnancy

Do you feel reassured that having 'periods' on the pill is not important? As discussed on p.40. | —YES→ | ● Continue taking same pill |

NO

● Discuss: probably best to move to a phased pill *or* up the ladder to a higher-dose pill

Very important: If only one 'period' missed and there is no reason to suspect failure of the pill, do not delay – start the next cycle of pills on the usual day (see page 53).

Fig. 17b Which pill? Bleeding patterns

who tends to have high blood levels a stronger pill than the lowest available – which would be more than enough for her! Those with low levels should still receive adequate protection against pregnancy, but will be prone to problems with the bleeding pattern. These can be managed, like other side-effects, by *forewarning*, and by following the scheme which I am about to describe.

Before we start examining this scheme, please read the footnotes to Figure 16 and bear in mind the need to be tactful and to DISCUSS the next move each time with your doctor.

Which pill to start with?

As just explained, the normal first choice these days should be the very lowest dose available from the selected progestogen ladder of Figure 15. But this rule must be applied flexibly (page 171). In particular, some women know themselves to be forgetful. Others will not tolerate or will become confused by *any* irregular bleeding. These may well be better off if given a slightly stronger brand from the outset (though normally still below the second line).

Commonly the first choice will prove satisfactory, long term. A given brand should normally be given at least two months' trial –

see Figures 16 and 17a. But if symptoms are troublesome come back as soon as necessary to discuss the next move:

If the first pill does not suit, which should be the second choice?

(a) *Problems with the bleeding cycle – bleeding on days of pill-taking.* Please look at Figure 17a and follow the questions and suggestions down the left-hand side. If you started taking the pill just after an abortion or miscarriage, the bleeding could have a special cause and you should turn at once to page 48. Otherwise one reason for this so-called 'breakthrough' bleeding is that there is too low a level of pill hormones in your blood, and therefore too little is reaching the lining of the uterus. It could also mean that there is too little for the contraceptive actions of the pill, and if you have been late in taking pills recently, or had a stomach upset, then you should follow the rules in Figures 11 and 12 (pages 50, 54–5). See also the text that goes with the figures, and pages 56–8 if there is the possibility that another drug is interfering with the pill's actions.

If you are only taking the first or second packet of pills, it is well worth persevering as improvement can be expected. Otherwise – and whenever bleeding is a persistent or unexplained problem, or occurs after love-making – you should see your doctor soon. There are some rare gynaecological causes for bleeding which he needs to eliminate by examining you. One example would be a polyp at the entrance to the uterus. Erosions (page 102) can very occasionally cause some kind of bleeding too. Any treatment necessary should be simple and minor, often just as an out-patient. But usually there is no gynaecological explanation. The problem can then often be solved by using a phased pill, pages 168–71; or otherwise by moving up the ladder to another pill which contains the same hormones as the one which you are presumably finding satisfactory in other ways. For example, if you were to develop 'breakthrough' bleeding or spotting with Ovysmen or Brevinor in ladder B your doctor might suggest Norimin. If necessary you could go up more rungs on the same ladder to Norinyl-1 or Ortho-Novin 1/50.

(b) *Problems with the cycle – no bleeding during the pill-free week.* You should now refer to Figure 17b. Have you forgotten any pills? Or has something else happened recently which might reduce your protection against pregnancy? If there is any doubt pregnancy must be ruled out by one or perhaps a series of urine tests and probably an examination (see page 53). If you start getting symptoms such as nausea or miss two periods in a row it is essential to have a pregnancy test even if you have been very good at taking your tablets.

Once the explanation of pregnancy has been ruled out, then you may like to stop and think whether it really bothers you whether you get bleeding between packets of pills or not. The fact is that no pill-user ever has real *periods* anyway. The bleeding which you think of as a period is entirely artificial (page 38) and caused by you when you stop taking pills for 7 days in each 28 days. If the loss of the pill hormones does not cause a bleed, it just means there was no blood to come away. So far as we know either no bleeding, or the passing of a little dark-brown discharge rather than blood, mean nothing as far as your health is concerned; and nor do they indicate any risk to your future fertility (see page 109). In fact, if you were to transfer to another method, I can almost guarantee that your periods would come back with no more delay than the average pill-user.

If this reassures you, you could, if you wish, stay on the same pill more or less indefinitely. Otherwise the solution once again, with the approval of your doctor, may be to try a phased pill. If that is unsatisfactory the brand on the next available rung up your particular ladder in Figure 15 will usually cause better bleeding during the pill-free days.

What about other side-effects which are nothing to do with the bleeding pattern?

Please refer now to the bottom half of Figure 16. If you have a symptom which could perhaps be serious (see the list on page 61), or if you are not sure that it is not one of those, you should contact your doctor today and take no further pills unless the doctor says that you may. If it is a less serious side-effect such as gain in weight, headaches which are not migraines, or breast symptoms; and if it continues beyond the two or three courses of pills which are necessary to give your body a chance to get used to any particular brand, then there are two possibilities. First, if you are currently taking a pill from above the lower line in Figure 15, this might be a good time to discuss a move down the

177

ladder to a pill below that line. Otherwise, you could move further down your current ladder provided there is a pill brand available which contains even less hormone. NB *Always follow the rules on page 59 if going down a ladder.*

If there is no room for you to go down any more rungs on a particular ladder, or it seems possible that your side-effect is due to a particular progestogen, then the other possibility to discuss with your doctor is a 'sideways shift'. This means moving to a different ladder altogether and taking a pill which contains a different progestogen combined with the oestrogen. It would still be best to take the lowest possible total dose of hormones. There are some guidelines which may sometimes be helpful in deciding which of the two hormones in the pill is the one whose dose should be lowered the most:

(a) *Conditions linked with relative oestrogen excess may be helped by a more* PROGESTOGEN-DOMINANT *pill*
nausea
dizziness
symptoms of tension/irritability
feelings of bloating/cyclical weight gain due to fluid retention
vaginal discharge (no infection present)
some cases of breast tenderness with enlargement
growth of breast lumps (page 114)
growth of fibroids (page 104)
endometriosis (page 105)

For any of these problems (a) it is often worth trying a progestogen-dominated pill – i.e. one with the lowest possible dose of oestrogen combined with *relatively* more progestogen. Lowering the oestrogen (e.g. Loestrin 20, but see comment on page 174) is usually preferable to raising the progestogen (as in Eugynon 30/Ovran 30), for the reasons discussed on pages 131–3. Loestrin 30 might be the first choice here.

(b) *Conditions linked with relative progestogen excess may be helped by a more* OESTROGEN-DOMINANT *pill.*
some cases of sustained weight gain
some cases of depression/tiredness
loss of sex urge (libido)
dryness of vagina
acne, and greasiness of skin and head hair
unwanted hair growth (hirsutism)

For these problems (b) the most oestrogen-dominant pills are the first ones *above the top line* in each of the ladders C, D, E and F. Severe acne needs 50 mcg oestrogen for best results. But, on the general principle of lowering the total dose of hormone given, among the ultra-low combined pills the most oestrogen-dominant formulae are Ovysmen/Brevinor and Logynon/Trinordiol.

Another possibility would be desogestrel pills (page 168). Desogestrel is believed to be less androgenic (page 168); and that tendency may explain most side-effects due to other progestogens. There is also available in some countries under the brand name Diane a pill containing a particular progestogen with strong anti-androgenic effects in the body, cyproterone acetate, combined with 50 mcg of ethinyloestradiol. This is recommended chiefly for the *treatment* of severe acne and hirsutism, but it is also an effective contraceptive.

Fortunately, most women find the first pill they try is satisfactory.

Are all side-effects actually caused by the treatment received?

In one very interesting research study from Mexico, 147 women who had recently had a miscarriage and did not mind too much when they again became pregnant were given tablets which they thought were some kind of contraceptive. In fact, however, they were all given nothing more than *placebos* (dummy tablets of milk-sugar plus starch). These 147 women were then followed for a total of 424 woman-months. During only one-third of these months of observation were there no symptoms reported. Decreased libido was reported in 30 per cent of these months; dizziness 11 per cent of the time; indeed no less than 31 different effects of the 'no treatment' were reported!

Similar results were obtained in studies in which the pill was compared with dummy tablets without the women knowing which they were receiving. (They were using another method as their contraceptive.) Other studies in which placebo tablets were used in comparison with other drugs, and where the volunteers were men, have similarly shown that dummies can 'cause' numerous symptoms.

The reason for referring to this research is not to say women imagine the problems they have with the pill, which can be real enough as already described in this book. However it must be clear that the pill could sometimes be blamed for things which are not really caused by any effects of its hormones. If women are very anxious about possible health risks of taking the pill, or if their doctor or nurse is in a hurry and fails to inspire them with any confidence, it seems that they are more likely to complain of such problems as dizziness, headaches, and mild depression. On the other hand, researchers have shown that women who do not often complain of nervous symptoms, or who are prescribed the pill by somebody who answers their questions and is reassuring and checks by examining them that all is well, are much less likely to complain of symptoms from the pill, to keep changing brands, or to discontinue it altogether.

In the RCGP Study no less than 27 per cent of the pill-users stopped the method in the first year while still feeling the need for contraception. No fewer than 199 symptoms or diseases were given as the reason for giving up the pill, and in only a small fraction is there any convincing evidence of them being a true effect of the pill. A further very relevant fact is that about one in five of these women who stopped the pill while still planning to continue avoiding pregnancy in fact became pregnant within the next year. Perhaps more should have considered:

The mini-pill or progestogen-only pill

This is the place to look in detail at this pill which contains no oestrogen at all. It can be a logical choice especially:

(i) if reducing the health risk of your method to the absolute minimum is particularly important to you;

(ii) if you are a woman with a relative contra-indication to the combined pill from the list on page 155;

(iii) if you have a side-effect problem which has not been dealt with by following the suggestions of Figure 16.

Turn to the next chapter and the secrets of this increasingly popular kind of pill will be revealed.

8

The progestogen-only pill (mini-pill)

What are mini-pills?

First let us be clear what they are not. They are not low-dose combined pills, which have been the subject of most of this book so far. It is very confusing that two of these start with 'Min' (i.e. Minovlar and Minilyn). Even ultra-low-dose combined pills still contain both the hormones oestrogen and progestogen.

Because the word 'mini-pill' causes so much confusion, I shall just label them progestogen-only pills or POPs for short.

Unlike combined pills, POPs are taken every day while contraception is needed including during periods. They contain no oestrogen and the progestogen itself is generally also in a lower dose than in combined pills. So it is believed that they are even less likely to harm your health than combined pills. Note carefully that though this is a reasonable belief, it has not been *proved* true. POPs have not been used by enough women for long enough for the possible medium- to long-term unwanted effects to show up. Over all they have not yet been studied nearly as thoroughly as the combined pills. However, it is known that, like them, an overdose of POPs can cause no serious harm to an average adult or child.

How do they work?

You will find it helpful to refer to Table 10. It shows that POPs do not depend on stopping release of the egg. As a result, most periods that a woman gets on this pill, unlike those on the combined pill (page 38), are natural ones. They are due to the loss of the natural progesterone and oestrogen from the ovary

Table 10 How progestogen-only pills prevent pregnancy
(The more +s means the greater the effect)

	'Ordinary' combined pills	Progestogen-only mini-pills
1. Reduced FSH therefore follicles stopped from ripening and egg from maturing	++++	+
2. LH surge stopped so no egg-release	++++	++
3. Cervical mucus changed into a barrier to sperm	+++	+++
4. Lining of uterus made less suitable for implantation of an embryo	+++	++(+)
5. Uterine tubes perhaps affected so that they do not transport egg so well (uncertainty about this)	+	+
Expected pregnancy rate per 100 women using the pill method for one year (compare use of NO METHOD = 80–90)	0.1–1	0.5–4

Notes:
The combined pill is *very* reliable with plenty of back-up effects – but relies chiefly on effects 1 and 2.
The progestogen-only pill relies chiefly on effects 3 and 4. Egg-release is disturbed or stopped in about half of all POP-users, increasingly with increased duration of use.

reaching the lining of the uterus, as the corpus luteum comes to the end of its usual limited life span – about two weeks after egg-release.

So POPs operate by interfering with the passage of sperm through the mucus at the entrance to the uterus (cervix). The slippery mucus which is normally released under the influence of oestrogen is altered by the artificial progestogen and becomes a scanty and thick material which is an effective barrier to the sperm. This happens whether or not the POP prevents egg-release that month. One way of looking at this is to *consider the POP as a barrier method of family planning which is taken by mouth.*

The most important of the other changes which help to prevent pregnancy, shown in Table 10, are those that affect the lining of the uterus. The progestogen of the POP acts directly on it, perhaps altering its special receptors for hormones. It often affects the lining indirectly by interfering with the corpus luteum so that its natural progesterone production is reduced. Both these effects seem to make the lining of the uterus less suitable for implantation of an embryo: even if a sperm did manage to get through the mucus barrier. It is possible that transport of the egg by the uterine tubes is also impaired, so that it dies before or after fertilization and before implantation can occur.

How effective are POPs?

If taken very regularly they are capable of giving protection second only to the combined pill. The failure rate is about 0.5–4 per 100 woman-years. See page 38 for what this means. Much depends on the efficiency of the user and how fertile she is. The lower figure applies to older women (over 35–40) for whom this can be a most reliable method and roughly amounts to an 'evens chance' of one pregnancy after 200 years. But of course that one pregnancy could happen in the first year rather than the last.

This pill is therefore usually more suitable for older than for young and highly fertile women. You should discuss the pros and cons with your doctor.

How are POPs taken?

The answer is: every single day, 365 days a year, at the same time of day, and whether or not you are having any kind of bleeding that day. In the last chapter I pointed out that the ultra-low-dose combined pills of Table 8 (page 162) are very effective but may have a slightly reduced margin for error. This is even more true of the progestogen-only pills. They can be at least as reliable as an IUD, and perhaps more so if taken with the regularity of clockwork; preferably at exactly the same time each day – and best of all at around 6 or 7 o'clock in the evening.

When should POPs be taken?

The sperm-barrier effect on the cervical mucus mentioned just now reaches its maximum about four or five hours after each

183

pill is taken. As the commonest time for love-making is around bedtime, the very best time to take this pill is in the early evening, say at 7 o'clock. This is not to say that if you fancy sex at breakfast-time or in the middle of the afternoon you will not be protected. Once you are fully established on the POP you should have quite adequate protection at any time in the 24 hours. It is just logical to have the best possible protection around the most common time for your own love-making. There could of course be problems if your partner is on night-duty or if you are: you just have to work things out between you!

This argument means that *for most women the very worst time to take their POP is bedtime* because they are then regularly relying on the mucus effect from the pill taken 24 hours earlier. So pill-taking at breakfast or lunch-time would be better and indeed perfectly acceptable. More important than the precise time is the regularity with which you take your pill at the same hour of each day. Yet it is not as reliable as the combined pill, so no one can promise you *complete* security against pregnancy even if you are obsessionally regular in your pill-taking.

How do I start taking this pill?

You take your first tablet on the first day of *your next period*, and start each subsequent packet immediately following the last tablet of the previous one. Because the full effects shown in Table 10 take some time to build up, it is suggested that you do not rely on this pill until you have taken it for fourteen days. This means using a method like the sheath during that time – though this might be too cautious, see Important Note, page 185.

No extra precautions are required if the POP is started on the day of a *miscarriage* or *termination of pregnancy*.

After *delivery of a baby*, this pill does not increase the risk of blood clots. So it can be started as early as the seventh day. No extra precautions are required, either then or if you prefer to delay starting the POP until the fourth week after the birth. This applies even if you do not breast-feed.

Another option: if periods have not yet returned, start the POP any time, but allow at least one week before unprotected intercourse occurs.

From and to the combined pill

1. *From the combined pill to the POP*. Take the first pill from the POP packet the day after the last combined pill. As there is some 'carryover' of the latter's contraceptive effects, it is then probably unnecessary to use another method for the first fourteen days of POP-taking.

2. *From the POP to the combined pill,* or another family planning method. It is best to have the first packet of the combined pill ready, and to transfer directly to it on the first or second day of your next definite period, perhaps before you have finished the final POP packet. This is also the best time to stop if you are transferring to a method like the sheath or the cap. The reason is that waiting to the end of your POP packet might coincide with egg-release, at the most fertile time two weeks before the next period – not a good time for changing methods.

If you do not see any periods (see below) then you could wait until the end of your current packet before taking the first combined pill, or starting another new method. Either way you can assume continuous protection against pregnancy.

What if I forget to take a POP?

This pill is not for the forgetful. The rules are stricter than with the combined pill. Please study Figure 18 carefully.

If you are more than *3 hours* late in taking the pill, then you should take the one you have missed but use another method for fourteen days after the pill was forgotten. Should you have an *attack of diarrhoea*, or *vomit* within 3 hours of pill-taking and be unable to keep another pill down within the 3 hours, similar loss of protection must be assumed.

Important Note: The 14-day part of the rule just given is being very much questioned. The most important contraceptive effect, on the mucus (Table 10), takes only a few hours to build up, and the others are probably adequate within a couple of days. Personally I therefore favour a 2-day rule, and hope this will be officially recognized before the next edition of *The Pill*.

The effectiveness of the POP can be regained quickly: but there is no doubt that it is less than that of the combined pill, and it is also *losable much more rapidly – within 3 hours, in fact*. No change there.

What about interactions between the POP and other medicines?

The POP has never been widely enough used for us to be able to answer some of the questions about it – and this is one of them. However, to be on the safe side, we have to assume that *with the exception of antibiotics*, those medicines that can affect the combined pill also reduce the effectiveness of the mini-pill. See the discussion on pages 56–8 and Table 2a. So the POP is not reliable enough against pregnancy when used, for example, by women with epilepsy who have to be on a drug from Table 2. It seems unlikely, however, that the opposite effect is true: in other words, the POP probably does not interfere with the action of other medicines to any important extent.

In all these circumstances – missing pills, stomach upsets (vomiting or diarrhoea), the use of interfering drugs – your loss of protection against pregnancy is more likely and more immediate than with the combined pill. You are also more likely to get irregular bleeding which is in any case a commoner problem on the POP.

What if I am late for a period?

As a general rule on this pill, whatever your periods do, coming early or late, or not at all, do not stop taking the tablets unless advised to do so by a doctor. Irregular bleeding and no bleeding are the main side-effects. But if you go six weeks with no period, and especially if you see no bleeding during the four weeks after pills have been missed or after a stomach upset, you do need to arrange a pregnancy test on an early morning specimen of your urine, to be on the safe side. See again Figure 18. It is especially important to arrange this test and see your doctor if you get symptoms like early morning nausea. If the result is negative you should take your doctor's advice as to whether and how often it should be repeated: no need of course if you then get a period. If the test shows you are pregnant you should stop taking the pill. If pregnancy is extremely likely because you have missed more than one pill while taking no other precautions (see Figure 18), your doctor may well advise you at an earlier stage to stop the method. In fact the tiny dose of progestogen in the POP is even less likely than the ordinary pill to harm an early pregnancy (see page 110). But it is better to play safe, using another kind of contraception until you know for sure.

What if I continue with no periods and am shown not to be pregnant?

This is rather more complicated. In some women, even the small amount of hormone present in the POP can be enough to stop egg-release. This means two things: first, the base of the brain and pituitary gland are being made inactive by this low dose of a single hormone in the same way as happens in any woman who is taking any 'ordinary' combined pill. *So no egg-release means you are as protected against pregnancy as if you were on the combined pill.* But second, *on the progestogen-only pill, no egg-release means no periods.* Why not? The reason of course is that on the POP you do not *(and must not)* take the pills in a cyclical way, with the regular 7-day break in each 28 days. That is what causes the 'periods' on the ordinary pill (see page 38). They are quite artificial, caused by the pill hormones acting directly on the lining of the uterus, and should really be called 'hormone withdrawal bleeds'.

If then you get no periods at all on the POP no eggs are being released: so you are actually much better protected from pregnancy than any friend of yours also using this pill who goes on seeing regular periods and is therefore being continually reassured!

Of course this is only true if you continue to be unfailingly regular in taking your pills, and even then only if tests and perhaps an examination have proved that the method has not let you down. It is a bit muddling that the same situation – i.e. absence of periods – could mean *either* that you are already pregnant *or* that you are extra safe against pregnancy! It can also be rather worrying and is one of the problems of the POP method. As usual, if in doubt, discuss the next step with your doctor.

How reversible is the POP?

As the dose of hormone is so low, the fertility of a woman after stopping this pill is believed to be the same as it would have been

187

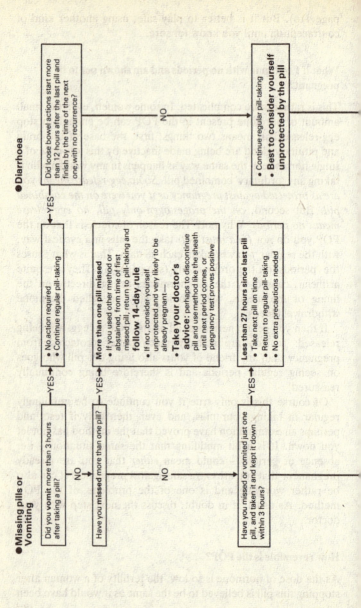

● Diarrhoea

Did loose bowel actions start more than 12 hours after the last pill and finish by the time of the next one, with no recurrence?

NO →
- Continue regular pill-taking
- **Best to consider yourself unprotected by the pill**

YES ↓

- No action required
- Continue regular pill-taking

● Missing pills or Vomiting

Did you **vomit** more than 3 hours after taking a pill?

YES →
- No action required
- Continue regular pill-taking

NO ↓

Have you **missed** more than one pill?

YES →

More than one pill missed
- If you used other method or abstained, from time of first missed pill, return to pill-taking and **follow 14-day rule**
- If not, consider yourself unprotected and very likely to be already pregnant—
- **Take your doctor's advice:** perhaps to discontinue pill and use method like the sheath until next period comes, or pregnancy test proves positive

NO ↓

Have you missed or vomited just one pill, and taken it and kept it down within 3 hours?

YES →

Less than 27 hours since last pill
- Take next pill on time
- Return to regular pill-taking
- No extra precautions needed

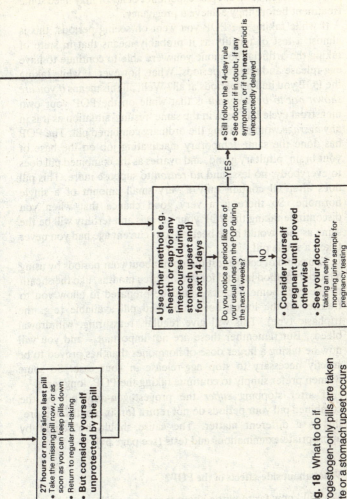

27 hours or more since last pill
- Take the missing pill now, or as soon as you can keep pills down
- Return to regular pill-taking
- **But consider yourself unprotected by the pill**

- **Use other method e.g. sheath or cap for any intercourse (during stomach upset and) for next 14 days**

Do you notice a period like one of your usual ones on the POP during the next 4 weeks?

YES →
- Still follow the 14-day rule
- See doctor if in doubt, if any symptoms, or if the next period is unexpectedly delayed

NO →
- **Consider yourself pregnant until proved otherwise**
- **See your doctor**, taking an early morning urine sample for pregnancy testing

Fig. 18 What to do if progestogen-only pills are taken late or a stomach upset occurs

Note: The 14-day rule is the official rule – but is under discussion. See Important Note, page 185.

189

at her age if she had never taken it. Remember though that at least one in ten of all couples experience delay or may need some treatment before they achieve a pregnancy.

If while taking the POP you went on seeing periods, this is almost a test of fertility as it probably means that in spite of taking the artificial hormone you were able to continue to have egg-release and natural periods. What, however, if while taking the POP you had no periods at all? Well, all this means *if you are shown not to be pregnant* is that while on the POP your own menstrual cycle has been in the same 'resting' situation as it is in any *average* woman taking the ordinary combined pill. The POP has done the same temporary inactivating job on the base of your brain, pituitary gland, and ovaries as the combined pill does to everybody: no less, and *no reason* to suppose more. This pill does after all contain only a very small amount of a single hormone. So there is a very good chance that when you discontinue taking the POP your periods and fertility will be the same as they would have been at your current age had you never taken a single pill.

You could of course test the point about your periods by using a barrier method instead for two or three months, like the sheath or the cap. Some doctors would be prepared to allow you to transfer to the lowest-dose combined pill available (e.g. the triphasic type). This will give regular, reassuring, withdrawal bleeds. But remember these are not important – and you will now be taking a larger dose of hormones than has proved to be strictly necessary to stop egg-release in your case. So some women prefer simply to continue taking the POP, long term.

If after stopping *either* the progestogen-only pill *or* the combined pill your periods do not return for six months or more, this is a different matter. The cause should be sought by appropriate examinations and tests (see page 63).

What about side-effects of the POP?

We still know far too little about these, especially any long-term effects, but what we do know is reassuring when compared with our knowledge about the combined pill.

* Research into *body chemistry* has come up with different results from that on the combined pills. The factors involved in blood clotting seem to be quite unaffected on the POP. They also return to normal if a woman transfers to it from the combined pill. But the Glucose Tolerance Test mentioned on page 74 is minimally changed in POP-users, and there are slight changes in the blood levels of the hormone insulin and in blood fats (lipids). Some studies suggest that these are actually even less affected by some 'bottom-of-the-ladder' combined pills in Figure 15 (page 165). In other words the oestrogen in those can cancel out some of the effects of the progestogen on body chemistry, as discussed on page 132. But the same oestrogen has other snags which are well established (especially its effects on clotting factors). So the picture is confused at present. All one can say is that the relative advantages of the POP over the lowest-dose available combined pills may not be as great as was once thought even as recently as the first edition of this book.

Blood pressure can be a little bit higher during POP-taking than it is when no hormone is taken. Over all, however, blood pressure tends to be *much* less affected than on the combined pill. It often falls on transferring from the combined pill to the POP.

In general the systems of the body seem to be affected less by this pill than even the lowest-dose combined pills in Figure 15.

So the POP is an excellent pill and would be much more widely used if only it did not tend to cause an *erratic bleeding pattern*. Although the periods which happen are caused the normal way (page 181), the progestogen can, and often does, modify a POP-user's cycle, and affect the bleeding mechanisms of the lining of the uterus. So, on the one hand, as already explained, there may be complete absence of bleeding for months on end. On the other hand, periods can be more frequent; longer or shorter than before; very irregular; or relatively regular with frequent and unexpected extra bleeds from the lining of the uterus in between the periods. This is the major problem of the method. But forewarned is forearmed and many women adjust very well after a month or two to their new bleeding pattern. Other symptoms of the menstrual cycle, such as pre-menstrual tension, are very variable, depending on how much the cycle is altered by the POP. They are usually unchanged but in different women they can be worsened or improved!

A much smaller proportion of women than is found on the combined pill complain of things like *weight gain, loss of libido, acne, breast tenderness, headache,* and *dizziness*. As with the combined pill, these symptoms are usually only a problem in the first two or three months and it is worth persevering at least that long as they could well disappear. A few women also complain of pain caused by *cysts on the ovary* of the type described on page 106, though more often such cysts give no symptoms. Far from protecting against these as the combined pill does, the POP actually makes them more likely to be formed.

Finally, like the IUD, if a pregnancy does occur during use of the POP it seems it may be more likely to be in the wrong place: particularly in the uterine tube. This is known as an *ectopic pregnancy*. This is a rare complication, occurring in about 1 in 1,000 POP-users per year in a country like Britain: but it is serious as the pregnancy cannot continue normally. Eventually it may break into a blood-vessel. As this could lead to internal bleeding an emergency operation is essential.

A possible explanation is that egg-release can still occur; a sperm may manage to get through the barrier of altered cervical mucus; and then because of the slowing-down effect of progestogen on the normal functioning of the tube, the fertilized egg may get held up and grow there rather than on the wall of the uterus. In practice, this means that if while on the POP you start to have an increasingly severe pain in the lower abdomen, usually on one side or the other, and not coming and going like normal menstrual cramps, then you should be seen and *examined* by a doctor. If the cause is an ectopic, the period will generally be a few days overdue, or you may have had what seemed like a prolonged and lighter-than-usual period. However, even without this, when in doubt you should see your doctor promptly. If he or she feels it possible that you have a pregnancy in the tube – it can often be very difficult to be sure – then you will be referred to the nearest hospital for further tests and possibly an operation if required.

Who should avoid the POP?

At present there is some uncertainty about this. The simple and generally accepted policy followed by many doctors is to avoid the POP in all the conditions listed on pages 149–55 which were described as reasons for never taking the combined pill. Although there is no research that proves that diseases of the circulation occur on the POP any more often than among non-users of any pill, a past history of any of these is still described as a reason for not taking them. But many doctors disagree with this policy and are prepared to use the POP for women who have such a past history, especially if it concerned a venous – not arterial – thrombosis. But this would only be after full discussion and with careful medical supervision.

An extra reason for avoiding the POP would be any history of an ectopic pregnancy – see above. As that rare complication reduces fertility (and also because of the higher failure rate of POPs, page 183), younger women who want a family in due course are normally advised to take the combined pill as first choice over the POP. But the latter is still a good second choice for many.

Since it contains no oestrogen, the POP does not usually have to be stopped during immobilization or before major surgery.

Which variety of POP should I choose?

The kinds available in Britain are as shown in Table 11, and also in Figure 15 in the last chapter, where they are shown as at 'ground level', because they contain so little hormone. If you live in another country, refer again to the World Directory of pill names (page 266) to discover how the locally available brands of POP are related to those shown here.

Any of these pills may prove satisfactory. If you develop a problem with the cycle or any other side-effect with one POP, and still wish to use the method, then it is certainly worth switching to one of the others. At the moment this has to be done very much on a trial-and-error basis. If you persevere, the menstrual pattern normally becomes acceptable after a few months. If you get no periods at all, and this is shown not to be due to pregnancy, there is often no medical objection to your continuing the same POP. Group A (levonorgestrel) pills usually allow the period to happen, and are also the best to try if there is

193

* **Table 11** Brands of progestogen-only pills available in Britain

Name of pill	No. in packet	Progestogen content (milligrams)	Remarks
Group A			
Neogest	35	levonorgestrel 0.0375	Plus in addition 0.0375 mg of *inactive* progestogen
Microval	35 ⎫	levonorgestrel 0.03	⎰ No extra, inactive, hormone –
Norgeston	35 ⎭		⎱ these are therefore preferred to Neogest
Group C			
Micronor	42 ⎫	norethisterone 0.35	
Noriday	28 ⎭		
Group E			
Femulen	28	ethynodiol diacetate 0.5	

Note: Groups A, C, E contain the same progestogens as the groups with the same letter in Tables 8 and 9 (pages 162, 163) and the ladders in Figure 15 (pages 165–7).

a blood pressure problem. But if bleeding becomes excessive it may be worth discussing with your doctor the possibility of transferring to one of the slightly higher-dose POPs from the Table.

Who might consider using the POP?

The short answer is, anyone who is considering taking a pill at all. This would be the obvious choice if maximum safety against health risk is particularly important to you. You will be losing a bit in effectiveness as compared with the combined pill: but not too much if you are good at remembering to take pills, especially if you are over 35 (page 183). A lot may depend on how well you manage to live with an unpredictable menstrual cycle.

Because of these two snags, the POP really comes into its own when there is a *relative contra-indication* to the combined pill. This means the second list on pages 155–60 of *conditions which require special supervision* if any pill is taken. (But as noted on page 186, item 11 on that list, the long-term use of 'interfering' drugs, would usually go against the choice of a POP.)

Out of the list, I think the POP is particularly valuable for *smokers* and for *women over the age of 35* (page 157). It is excellent for *diabetics*, both because it seems to cause less health risk and because it is extra effective as they can remember to

194

take it so regularly with their evening insulin injection. This is the best time of day (page 183). It can be tried sometimes with success in those with *blood pressure problems* on the pill. It may also be recommended if you have a history of *irregular periods* or times in the past, before having taken any hormones, when you had no periods at all for many months. It is of course then very likely that you will have no periods at all on the POP; but if you can put up with that it is probably true that this variety of pill causes least suppressing effect on the base of your brain and the pituitary gland. Some doctors recommend the POP for women *nearing the change of life*.

So far as we know this is fine, but it should be used with caution for the following reasons: firstly, we are still unable to be certain that the additional risk of heart attacks and strokes which all women at this age run will not be increased, slightly, especially in smokers, by progestogens even in the small dose used in POPs. There is also the same uncertainty as with the combined pill about the possible effects of duration of use (pages 126–30, though they should be even less, if they exist at all, with the tiny dose used in POPs.

Secondly, if the POP-user has no periods, it can be quite difficult to know when the menopause actually happens, though a blood test can sometimes help. High values of the hormone FSH are to be expected if the menopause has occurred. Then the POP can be stopped and another method used for one year. If there is still no period, this is the classical way to decide that it is safe to have unprotected intercourse: but the wait can be shortened considerably if after stopping the POP a repeat FSH test is high in a woman over age 45.

Thirdly, if irregular bleeding occurs, particularly between periods, it may be necessary to do tests or perhaps a D & C, to be sure that there is no gynaecological problem.

Incidentally, so-called hormone replacement therapy, which may be prescribed for symptoms around the menopause, should not be relied on as a contraceptive. The dose system is different from that used in any kind of contraceptive pill, and pregnancy is possible – unless of course you had definitely reached the menopause, as defined above, before the treatment started.

If any of this applies to you and you have any queries, discuss the whole matter with your doctor or the clinic.

The commonest reason why many women choose to transfer to the POP is *because of side-effects* on the combined pill. Weight gain, nausea, depression, and headaches all seem to be helped by this move. Blood pressure has already been mentioned. If a combined pill-user develops chloasma, the skin pigmentation problem described on page 115, it often improves if she transfers to the POP.

Breast-feeding

This pill does not interfere at all with the quantity or significantly with the quality of breast milk. (The combined pill, however, sometimes does, and most doctors now feel that it is illogical to use it during breast-feeding.) A very tiny amount of the hormone in all POPs has been shown to get into the milk, the least being found in milk from women who use pills containing only levonorgestrel – i.e. Norgeston and Microval. This causes concern to some mothers. It is true that we really have no adequate knowledge of what effects the POP content of a mother's milk might have on the newborn baby. And yet, putting it the other way, there is absolutely no evidence that this amount of hormone has ever caused a baby any harm. After more than two years of full breast-feeding the infant of a mother using these POPs will have taken the equivalent of just one tablet!

To put this in perspective, if a breast-feeding woman smokes cigarettes, a far greater number of potentially dangerous chemicals are swallowed by the baby (see page 41).

If you plan to feed your baby yourself – and there is abundant scientific evidence that human breast milk is better for human babies than any kind of modified cow's milk – you might discuss the use of this type of pill during the months that you are breast-feeding. Your protection against pregnancy is probably as good as that of any woman on the combined pill, as *full* breast-feeding supplements the contraceptive action of the POP. When you or your baby decide to cut down on the breast-feeding, and especially when your periods return, you may well prefer to change back to an ultra-low-dose combined pill from Table 8, page 162. This will give extra reliability and a regular monthly 'period'. On the other hand, you may find that the POP is so satisfactory that you prefer to continue using it.

9

The future of family planning: and what became of the male pill?

It should by now be very clear that both types of pill discussed in this book leave a lot of room for improvement. What should we look for in an IDEAL future method of birth control?

Perhaps the last item in Table 12 which lists the features of the ideal contraceptive is asking for too much, but we *are* talking about the ideal! For all its faults, the pill does help women who suffer discomfort or misery from their so-called 'normal' menstrual cycles. A method which was ideal in all the main ten ways listed in the Table, such as a simple, painless, totally reversible method of female sterilization, might still leave some women less well off than on the pill, if they continued to have heavy, painful periods, pre-menstrual tension, and the like.

Table 12 Features of the ideal contraceptive

---

1. 100 per cent effective
2. 100 per cent safe, with no unwanted effects . . . { no danger / no nuisance
3. 100 per cent reversible
4. Independent of intercourse
5. Effective after acceptable, simple, painless procedure(s), not relying on the user's memory
6. Reversed by a simple, painless process
7. Cheap, based on simple technology, easy to distribute
8. Independent of the medical profession
9. Acceptable to every culture, religion, and political view
10. Used by, *or* obviously visible to, the woman . . . plus, as an *optional extra* –
   • Giving the user a genuine 'bonus' – one or more *good* side-effects!

I wish it were not necessary to add number 10 to the list, but I think the point should be made. It is a sad comment on the relationship of many couples that they can sleep together yet be unable to trust each other. More specifically, some men are not trustworthy about contraception. Others are just forgetful or careless. An advantage of the sheath is that it gives visual proof that it has in fact been effectively used. If a male pill were ever available, it is not difficult to believe there might be some men who would claim to be taking it when they were not. See also page 213.

A final and very important point to notice about the list is that if a future method could be devised which had all these features, it would make contraception just like conception: something entirely under the control of the couple concerned, which 'comes naturally', with no need to involve doctors or hopefully anyone else.

Why have we not yet got better methods of family planning?

This is a good question: part of the answer is that until the last fifteen years or so, too little money and scientific effort were put into this kind of work. Looking back it seems incredible, but family planning research did not seem to be important; and indeed at one time many people thought it was analogous to devising better methods of house-breaking, so sinful did they perceive birth control to be! See page 9. We have come a long way since then, in our attitudes to sex and the role of women. But there are other reasons too why we still do not have ideal methods. Generally, in medicine, one is treating an abnormal body process, caused by disease. In trying to find a method of birth control the main action is to interfere with a *normal* body process and this means taking extra-special care. The method will be used by initially healthy women or men and should not make them unhealthy; on the other hand, it could be used by people who are already unhealthy and must not do them additional harm. It will be used in both developing and 'over-developed' countries, and may pose special and different hazards in each situation. Reproduction is a very intricate mechanism, and unwanted effects have to be looked for in the offspring as well as in the user of the method. Finally, much important research cannot be done in humans for ethical reasons, yet the animals used for testing may differ in marked and sometimes misleading ways from humans.

One hopeful line of research therefore being followed is to study men and women who are otherwise healthy but known to be infertile. If their problem could be imitated in a reversible way this could provide some useful new methods. See also page 210.

This has been a difficult chapter to write. Sudden scientific breakthroughs could at any time render any list of future methods either obsolete or incomplete. What seems at the time of writing to be a promising lead, may prove in due course to be a blind alley: either because of unacceptable side-effects, or because of ineffectiveness when actually tested in human beings. So I would suggest you take more notice of general principles than of the few detailed examples there has been room to quote.

You will need to keep referring to Figure 19 which illustrates the various stages or events in reproduction at which birth control methods either now do, or one day could, operate. You will see that the various stages are numbered in the flow chart. The same numbers, within the symbols for maleness and femaleness, show where each particular process takes place on the two diagrams which illustrate male and female anatomy. The manufacture of sperm is followed by their maturing, in a very long coiled tube right beside the *testicle* known as the *epididymis*. It is only after going through this tube that the sperm are mature and able to swim vigorously to their goal. At ejaculation, the climax of intercourse, the sperm are conveyed along the *vas deferens* (vas). This process takes sperm to the base of the penis and then down the *urethra* which is the tube in the middle of the penis. From then on everything happens inside the body of the woman. The sperm have to travel from the top of the *vagina*, through the *cervix*, up through the cavity of the *uterus*, and into the *uterine tube*. Even though they matured in the epididymis, they still have not reached their full capacity for fertilizing an egg. The process called *capacitation* which finally prepares them for this occurs after the sperm get into the uterus. One only of these fully capacitated sperm enters and fertilizes the egg when they meet, usually about half-way along the tube.

You should find the rest of Figure 19 easy to follow as its

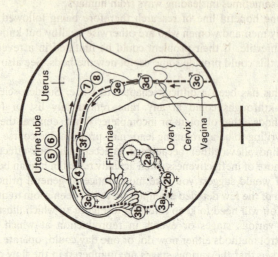

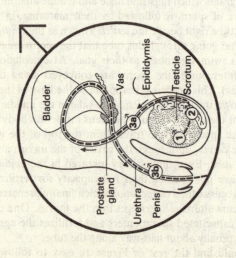

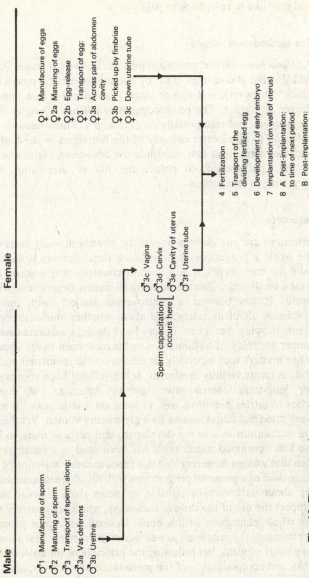

Male

♂1 Manufacture of sperm
♂2 Maturing of sperm
♂3 Transport of sperm, along:
♂3a Vas deferens
♂3b Urethra

Sperm capacitation occurs here ⎡ ♂3c Vagina
♂3d Cervix
♂3e Cavity of uterus
♂3f Uterine tube

Female

♀1 Manufacture of eggs
♀2a Maturing of eggs
♀2b Egg-release
♀3 Transport of egg:
♀3a Across part of abdomen cavity
♀3b Picked up by fimbriae
♀3c Down uterine tube

4 Fertilization
5 Transport of the dividing fertilized egg
6 Development of early embryo
7 Implantation (on wall of uterus)
8 A Post-implantation: to time of next period
   B Post-implantation: beyond next (missed) period

Fig. 19 The stages of reproduction

201

stages were described in Chapter 2, but if anything is not clear, you may like to refer back to pages 30–3.

The methods – in women

As I described earlier, combined pills work chiefly at stages ♀2a and ♀2b but also at stage ♂3d (by altering the cervical mucus to block the sperm), and also at stage 7 and possibly to a minor degree at stage 5. The progestogen-only pill has effects at the same stages, but relies chiefly on ♂3d and 7. Much research is going on to give better delivery of the hormones to the body, with two main aims: first, to reduce the dose given to the whole system, and second, to reduce the risk of user-failure by forgetting to take tablets.

Injections

Injections are one obvious possibility: already in many parts of the world a progestogenic drug called Depo-Provera is widely used for contraception, and in most countries it is used on at least a small scale. There is no room to discuss Depo-Provera in detail. It has become a controversial subject, with much discussion about its safety; and about whether animal experiments showing that it can, in very large doses, sometimes cause cancer are relevant to humans. Doubts have been raised about other matters too, especially its effects on the menstrual cycle and on future fertility in women. It has still not been approved for long-term contraceptive use in America, but many other countries permit its use, in some on a large scale. It has been 'tried and found *wanted*' by a great many women. Yet there are accusations that in the developed, and perhaps more so in the less developed countries, it has been used in a racist way; also that women have received this three-monthly injection of a large dose of a powerful progestogen without adequate counselling about its known or possible unknown risks. I would not support the use of the drug in such ways, which are contrary to the whole philosophy of this book. Nevertheless, some people are damning the drug itself as well as its incorrect use. It is a long way short of ideal, but following the principle of the balance of risks and acceptability – of the method, of alternatives, and of pregnancy – an individual informed woman may still feel that it is the best available option for her. It may be of positive benefit to some (e.g. sickle cell anaemia patients, page 151).

The main point about Depo-Provera is that it is a first faltering step along a road which both the consumers and the providers of family planning would find very acceptable. Many other compounds are now being tested, to be given by the injection route. They are mostly *progestogens*, the best known being Norigest (also known as Noristerat or Nur-Isterate). So far, like Depo-Provera, although highly effective against pregnancy, they tend to cause side-effects including such irregular bleeding that it is often dubbed 'menstrual chaos'. Tiny little polymer *microcapsules* are therefore being studied, which can be injected under the skin through an ordinary needle. It is hoped that they will give a more predictable slow release of the progestogen or other substance with which they are loaded.

One of the main problems of all injections is that they cannot be taken out once given, if side-effects occur. In an attempt to overcome that problem, experiments are being done with removable and re-loadable *implants*. One removable type is called Norplant. These are inserted and can if necessary be removed through small cuts in the skin.

Other contraceptive delivery systems

A variety of new ways to administer contraceptive substances to the body are being tried. *Pessaries* and *sponges* to be inserted into the vagina; *rings* around the cervix within the vagina; and even *contraceptive bracelets* tightly applied to the skin and *nasal sprays* are some of the ideas being studied.

The cervical rings release a progestogen, either alone or sometimes in combination with oestrogen, which is absorbed from the vagina. Contraception is achieved by some combination of the changes shown in Table 10, page 182, but with lower doses each day than in oral pills. All the woman has to do is to insert and remove her ring once a month or once every three months. Erratic bleeding is the main snag so far, but one version, sometimes given the name Varlevo-20, is just coming on the market in some countries.

Contraception through the nose is not such a fanciful idea as it

203

may sound at first: the chemists have been at work on the releasing hormone (RH) which conveys the message from the base of the brain to the pituitary to cause it to release FSH and LH (page 30). Various 'chemical cousins' (known as *analogues*) have been produced which when sprayed into the back of the nose do seem to be able to interfere with the action of the normal releasing hormone on the pituitary gland, and so prevent the stages ♀2a and ♀2b of Figure 19 – i.e. maturation and release of the egg.

A lot of research is also being devoted to using *intra-uterine devices* (IUDs) to convey certain drugs. So far these have chiefly been used in an attempt to reduce the side-effects of that method, particularly pain and increased bleeding. A promising version, which should soon be marketed, is the levonorgestrel-releasing IUD. This actually reduces menstrual bleeding, and differs from present IUDs in another way too: evidence suggests it *protects* against pelvic infection (compare page 221). The mechanism is probably similar to that described for progestogen-containing pills (the mucus effect, page 104). Another approach to avoiding those problems is to use *intra-cervical devices* (ICDs). These are experimental gadgets which fit inside the passageway of the cervix. They are designed to release either a progestogen or a spermicidal substance in a slow and steady way into the passage in order to prevent sperm going any further.

IUDs work mainly at stage 7 in Figure 19 by altering the interior of the uterus in such a way as to prevent the embryo from implanting. This was suspected for many years, but has been confirmed by doctors who have inserted IUDs up to five days after egg-release and found that even if the woman has had unprotected intercourse, she almost never becomes pregnant. This is therefore sometimes used now as a 'post-coital' or 'morning-after' method. Research goes on to learn how the IUD works in this way, leading hopefully to a method which produces the same effect without it being necessary to insert the foreign body at all.

New barrier methods

There is much interest again in these so-called 'old-fashioned' methods. A number of types of *sponges* are being tested, some made of synthetic polymers, some from natural collagen, some with and some without impregnation with standard or innovative spermicides. The *cervical cap* is also being re-examined and modified. It may be possible to design a plastic cap which exactly fits a particular woman's cervix. Provided with a one-way valve or similar mechanism to allow the exit of cervical mucus and the menstrual blood, it could perhaps be fitted and left in position for many months on end.

Post-coital contraception

This term can be used for any method which is first used after intercourse, and could act from stage ♀2b (if intercourse were known to have been prior to egg-release) right through to stage 8. Existing methods include *insertion of an IUD* as just described, or the use of high doses of *oestrogen* or a combination of *oestrogen and progestogen* (page 64). As they are used no more than 5 days (72 hours for the hormonal methods) after intercourse, they probably work chiefly at stage 7, implantation. Current methods are not recommended on a *regular* basis: however, other substances are now being examined which may prove safe for regular use.

'Once-a-month' methods

So the search is on for a method which causes the period to come on whether or not fertilization took place. Such *'once-a-month'* pills would be taken at the expected time of the period, and should be medically safer than daily pills because of the reduced dose. They all operate at stage 8A in the Figure. One group of substances being tested works by 'killing off' the corpus luteum, whose action is essential to prevent the next period washing an early pregnancy away. The same result could be obtained by interfering with the ability of the early pregnancy to maintain the corpus luteum by its hormone, hCG (page 29). This looks possible by both a drug method and an immune method described below.

These and other once-a-month approaches are being re-searched by the World Health Organization. As part of this programme of research it is looking at a number of plants which,

205

in various parts of the world, have gained the reputation for being contraceptive. One example is *Zoapatle*, which is used in Mexican folk medicine to produce periods. This and other chemicals derived from plants may well work chiefly by causing the uterus to contract vigorously, causing an early abortion. That is how *prostaglandins* work in humans, and partly explains why their early promise has not been fulfilled so far. Vigorous contractions of the uterus are painful, and there may also be other side-effects like vomiting and diarrhoea. However, it is hoped that chemical cousins of the prostaglandins – or derivatives of the plants just mentioned – may operate a few days earlier in the cycle and lead to a more normal period.

Methods working at or beyond the time of the first missed period (stage 8B)

If the IUD works largely by stopping implantation (stage 7) of an already fertilized egg, and if satisfactory once-a-month methods to work at stage 8A are devised, then obviously the dividing line between contraception and abortion is becoming increasingly blurred. However, stage 8B is clearly one of early abortion, and here the *prostaglandins* are already being used with some success. Because of the side-effects problem, there is no immediate prospect of a prostaglandin pill or vaginal pessary which the woman could safely use herself to produce a regular, very early abortion. There is an extra medical problem too and that is that the abortion might sometimes be incomplete. There would then be the risk of infection of the 'retained products' which could sometimes cause blockage of the uterine tubes, leading to infertility.

Ethical and moral aspects of methods operating after fertilization

Just as the definition of death has had to be altered – it is no longer cessation of the heartbeat, but death of the brain – so I think it is perhaps now out of date to say that methods which work after stage 4 (fertilization) are causing abortions. This is a very controversial area, but it seems to me that a lot of the arguments are just about definitions. I shall have to leave it to you to decide whether you do draw the line at stage 4; or else just

206

before or at the time of implantation (stage 7) which will allow you to consider the IUD, the POP (see effect 4 on page 182), and current post-coital pills as contraceptives. Points in favour of this view are: first, the *status* of the dividing fertilized egg, which is *100 per cent certainty of non-existence* unless it can stop the next menstrual flow by getting enough hCG to the ovary – and that requires implantation (page 29). Without 'carriage', how can one be 'procuring a miscarriage'? Secondly, is there logic in putting a high value on something with which nature itself is so prodigal (page 29)?

If doctors and patients are rather muddled on the subject, it is not surprising that the law in many countries is illogical and confused and the arguments often generate more heat than light! Perhaps the most important conclusion is that respect for life and a proper sense of awe at the whole process of reproduction are more important than rigid definitions.

Sterilization (stage ♂3f plus ♀3c)

If you refer to Table 12 (page 197) you will see that *female sterilization*, which prevents the sperm meeting the egg in the uterus tubes, could be ideal: if only it were even more simple and safe to perform, and if it were reversible. The latest methods of sterilization by applying clips or rings to block the tubes, often using a special telescope called the laparoscope, are already pretty good. Some surgeons have now become so skilled in microsurgery that they can join up the ends of the tube, after cutting away the short damaged section, and claim that 70 per cent of those re-operated on can have a baby. But this is not yet good enough: it is 'high technology' requiring much skill, and will be no help at all to poor people anywhere in the world.

The future may lie in some form of what is called *trans-cervical sterilization*. This means using the passageway that nature provided, through the canal of the cervix and the cavity of the uterus itself, in order to block the inner ends of the uterine tubes from within. Experiments have been carried out for some time now, with the aim of producing a cork or plug to be applied, and perhaps later removed, using another telescope instrument, the hysteroscope. Others are testing methods for applying special glues (which can stick tissues together) to the inner ends of the tubes, without using any special telescope. Even if not reversible, the prospect of doing such procedures in an out-patient clinic, with no more discomfort than the insertion of an IUD, is a welcome one – particularly for less developed countries. At the time of writing, however, there are still many technical problems.

* Immune methods

If a child is immunized against measles, an injection of a specially developed and less dangerous laboratory version of the virus causing measles is given. The child's body then produces *antibodies* which are actually special substances called immuno-globulins conveyed in the blood. The important point is that these are effective against *both* the laboratory virus *and* the natural one in the community which causes the disease. If that child is now exposed at school or anywhere to measles, the antibodies will destroy the virus. But the child can still get German measles or chicken pox, as the antibodies are, as it is called, *specific* against the one type of virus.

Now antibodies can be caused to appear not only against diseases, but also against any substances which are foreign to the body, *or* which can be altered in some subtle way so that the body treats them as though they were foreign. This can happen in an unwanted way to cause the so-called auto-immune diseases (page 119). But it also explains why it is theoretically possible to invent an immune method to work at many of the stages in Figure 19. Just one example: women could be made *immune to their husband's sperm*, and indeed this sometimes happens without being planned and causes one form of infertility. Some men develop *antibodies against their own sperm*, and although this does not always lead to them being infertile, it sometimes can do so. Again, this could lead to a male method.

There are many question marks about these methods, chiefly connected with the risk of complex antibodies being formed which might interfere with or injure other hormones, body chemicals, or tissues than those intended. However, one method, after an enormous amount of research, still appears quite promising, and is illustrated in Figure 20. The idea is to produce *a vaccine* which causes antibodies *against the hormone hCG* which was explained on pages 29, 32. This would stop the embryo 'rescuing' the corpus luteum, which it has to do if the

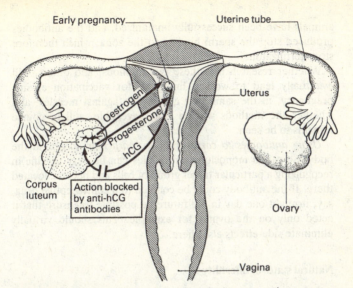

Fig. 20 The immune method: anti-hCG antibodies stop early pregnancy from maintaining corpus luteum

next period is to be prevented. If this worked, the method would lead to regular periods whether or not fertilization took place. The method might even be reversible, if the job of the corpus luteum of early pregnancy could be taken over by simply giving the woman the right dose of natural oestrogen and progesterone.

Depending on their definition of an abortion, some people would have genuine misgivings about the ethics of this. There has also been a serious technical problem in that as the antibody levels fall, female animals have tended to have later abortions rather than regular bleeds seemingly like normal periods. Abortions are bad news, not only ethically and psychologically, but also because of the risk of retained products, bleeding and infection.

* *Blocking fertilization (stage 4)*

To try to side-step these problems, researchers are now producing a vaccine whose target is the special covering of the egg known as the *zona pellucida*. This normally binds the sperm and allows just one in to fertilize the egg. Already laboratory

209

animals have been successfully immunized, and the antibodies produced stop the sperm binding to the zona, which therefore stops fertilizaton.

Whether research into these two methods, and others, will eventually lead to women lining up for vaccination against pregnancy, in the same way as they do against measles, and whether the methods will be truly reversible, still of course remains to be seen.

Using antibodies to carry drugs to 'particular' targets in the body. So-called monoclonal antibodies can be very specific in recognizing a particular target group of cells and become located there. If the antibody could be coupled to a contraceptive drug, say, it might one day in the future be possible to ensure that it acted only on the ovary, for example. This should virtually eliminate side-effects elsewhere.

Natural states of infertility

All women are unable to get pregnant at three main times in their lives: prior to puberty; in the earliest weeks of full breast-feeding, provided there is a very high frequency of suckling; and after the menopause. Forgetting the third state, for obvious reasons, the first two are being studied by scientists who hope to find out precisely what causes the lack of regular egg-release which prevents pregnancy at these times. A simple method of *making breast-feeding 100 per cent effective as a contraceptive*, which it certainly is not for most women for very long, would be most valuable for family spacing. Although the progestogen-only pill and the injection of Depo-Provera mentioned above can be used even now, they are open to the definite objection that some of the hormone (very much more in the case of Depo-Provera than the POP) gets into the breast milk, and could harm the baby in some as yet unknown way. A method which avoids this is obviously preferable.

Natural family planning (NFP)

It would be a major advance if a method could be devised which simply and accurately predicted beforehand, and detected afterwards, the release of the egg each month. This approach is acceptable to the Roman Catholic Church and certain other religious groups who do not accept methods which are 'artificial'. But in addition I think many other women and their partners would appreciate being able to use a simple method like the sheath or the cap just for the short time when they knew, because of some simple, accurate test, that there was a chance of pregnancy. Present methods depend on calculations according to the length of previous menstrual cycles; on taking and charting the early morning temperature; and on learning to recognize certain changes in the cervical mucus which usually occur before, during and after the fertile time. If the woman observes both mucus and temperature changes (the 'symptothermal' method), well-motivated couples can control their fertility well. The so-called *'intelligent thermometer'* now being tested should help, as the mini-computer it contains does all the decision-making, on the basis of daily temperature readings. But sooner or later many fertile long-term users even of the best existing natural family planning methods tend to be let down.

There are really two types of NFP method. One detects egg-release, and can be quite effective (because the egg dies quickly). The other tries to predict egg-release. This is obviously more difficult, but will always be less safe too: because of the *remarkably good and unpredictable survival of sperm* inside the uterus (see page 8).

Recently, *ultrasound scanning* – the same method that is used for checking the well-being of a baby as it grows in the uterus – has been used to watch the growth of the follicle on the active ovary, and to see the exact time of its rupture to release the egg. A really futuristic – and at present far too expensive – application of this method would be to issue women with mini-ultrasound-scan machines and teach them to observe their own egg-release!

More practical would be a simple test of the *saliva* or *urine*. The natural oestrogen and progesterone of the menstrual cycle are excreted in the urine in a modified form, and the changing levels of these excretory products can be measured. The end-result of this research should be that a woman could test her urine every day and, according to some easily interpreted colour change, she would know exactly when her unsafe period was. For instance, she could have intercourse from the first day

211

of her cycle just as long as the test showed 'green'. As soon as it changed to 'red', she would have to abstain or use another method. Whenever the test showed 'green' again, she could safely make love without any further precautions.

This research, which includes similar studies of saliva and of mucus, seems promising. It has the great advantage that the methods could be introduced without expensive and very time-consuming delays for safety testing which would be required for any new drug. But all these approaches are going to pose the problem that if they predict far enough ahead to allow for the most persistent surviving sperm, they may require an unpopular amount of abstinence by the couple.

New methods for men

'The latest development in male contraception was unveiled recently. Dr Sophie Merkin announced the preliminary findings of a study conducted on 763 male undergraduate students at a mid-West university.

The IPD (intra-penile device) resembles a tiny folded umbrella which is inserted through the head of the penis and pushed into the scrotum with a plunger-like instrument. Occasionally there is perforation of the scrotum, but this is considered insignificant since it is known that the male has few nerve endings in this area of his body.

Dr Merkin declared the IPD to be statistically safe for the human male. She reported that of the 763 students tested with the device, only two died of scrotal infection, only 20 experienced swelling of the tissues, three developed cancer of the testicles and 13 were too depressed to have an erection. She stated that common complaints ranged from cramping and bleeding to acute abdominal pains. She emphasized that these symptoms were merely indications that the man's body had not yet adjusted to the device. Hopefully the symptoms would disappear within a year.

One complication caused by the IPD and briefly mentioned by Dr Merkin was the incidence of massive scrotal infection necessitating the surgical removal of the testicles. "But this is a rare case", said Merkin, "too rare to be statistically significant". She and other distinguished members of the Women's College of

Surgeons agreed that the benefits far outweighed the risks to any man.'

OK: you've guessed, this IPD is a hoax. But there is nothing like a bit of role-reversal to throw new light on old arguments. In fact, of course, the pill and other methods of family planning for women are nowhere near as dangerous and frightening as this imaginary intra-penile device. Yet some overly enthusiastic family planners in the past have sometimes talked in the same *kind* of way about the pill for women. Hence the backlash: back in the early 1960s was the pill a confidence trick by male chauvinist scientists? Was there a conspiracy, with pharmaceutical companies keen to make money, to unleash an untried chemical on the unsuspecting, docile, and passive female population?

The main point is that 'what is sauce for the goose is sauce for the gander'. In other words, if we have a pill for the goose, we surely need a pill for the gander!

Do we need a male pill?

Some women doubt whether, if a safe and effective male pill were devised, men could be trusted to take it regularly. After all, they don't 'carry the baby'. There is a powerful concept in some parts of the world, known in Latin America as 'machismo', that – quite illogically in fact – equates fertility with virility and potency. These notions seem to have influenced researchers, who have wondered whether there would be a demand for a male pill even if it were invented.

Yet the assumption that men wash their hands of birth control matters is not in fact true. It takes all types to make a world and a great many men, especially in marriage or steady relationships, show a lot more responsibility than might perhaps be expected. The best example of this is the remarkable increase in the number of vasectomy operations performed in so many countries, both developing and developed, in recent years. Men, like women, now frequently prefer their families to be small. In one survey in America 65 per cent of the men stated that they would use a male pill or injection if it were available and not too expensive.

Research into male methods

Male contraception is biologically more difficult to achieve than female contraception. The main reason is that there is no single regular event like egg-release which can be stopped. See Figure 19. Stages ♂1 and ♂2 are continuous processes throughout a man's life from puberty to death. So instead of just stopping one egg being released about thirteen times a year, we have to interfere with a process producing hundreds of millions of sperm every time a man ejaculates. Just as in the woman, any pill must not affect libido, must give extremely good protection against pregnancy, and be as free as possible from side-effects. There is a special risk here too that interference with the production of the sperm might be incomplete. So one sperm might be damaged by whatever the treatment might be, and yet manage to fertilize an egg, leading perhaps to the birth of an abnormal baby.

Yet another problem is that the manufacturing process takes a long time, about seventy days in the human male. Thus any male pill working on the manufacturing process will take at least two months to become effective. It also means that there must be a long recovery period after stopping the method. After some of the experimental methods have been stopped, more than the usual number of abnormal sperm have been seen; and so if in the recovery period another method of family planning were inadequately used, again there might be an increased risk of an abnormal baby.

Interference with the manufacturing of sperm (stage ♂1)

This can be done in two main ways, indirectly by blocking the action of the hormones from the pituitary gland which normally stimulate the process, and directly by a drug acting on the testicles.

1. *Indirect methods.* These are similar in principle to the female pill. The pituitary gland of a man produces the very same two hormones that are so important in the menstrual cycle, namely FSH and LH. However, they are not produced in a cyclical way. In a man, FSH is the hormone which is directly involved to promote sperm manufacture. LH, on the other hand, stimulates special cells, also in the testicle, which produce the male hormone, testosterone. This hormone, as well as producing the

special sexual characteristics of a man such as the deepening of his voice, the hairiness of his chin, and his sex drive, joins with FSH in the business of manufacturing normal fertile sperm.

So if the levels of FSH and LH reaching the testicles can be made to drop, the process of sperm manufacture will cease. This can be done by 'negative feedback' which was explained on pages 31, 34. An obvious way of doing this is to feed the man with his wife's pill! This certainly cuts down the production of FSH and LH from the pituitary and hence interferes with manufacture of sperm. Obviously, however, it is liable to interfere also with the man's masculinity. One way out of that difficulty was to use a pill which is a combination of a *progestogen with an artifical equivalent of testosterone*. This has been promising but the doses required are relatively higher than in women and there are fears about serious unwanted effects, especially on the liver.

Other indirect methods are being tried, including the use of another hormone called *danazol*: or a complex natural substance called *inhibin*. There is also the possibility of blocking the action of RH which, as in a woman, comes down from the base of the brain to the pituitary gland and causes release of both FSH and LH. The same analogues of RH mentioned on page 204 are showing promise, used in the male in this way.

2. *Direct methods*. A bizarre approach has actually been tried, and that was to wrap the testicles up in warm, *woolly mufflers* made of sheepskin. This did lead to a drop in the sperm count because the sperm manufacturing process requires the testicles to be at a lower temperature than the 37 °C of the rest of the body. However, this method has not been found to reduce the count predictably enough to guarantee no pregnancies. There were also some complaints that it was uncomfortable.

Various drugs which directly damage the manufacturing process have been tried in male animals. The experiments have had to be abandoned in most cases because they were found to be too toxic.

One exception is *sulphasalazine*. This is a drug which has been used for years in the treatment of the disease ulcerative colitis, but only recently found to depress sperm counts enough to be considered for testing as a male pill. Another possibility is *gossypol*. A report on the use of this substance appeared in the

Chinese Medical Journal in November 1978. Scientific workers in Mainland China apparently discovered during the 1950s that cooking with crude cottonseed oil could lead to infertility, and it was the men that seemed to be affected. The active ingredient was tried first in a number of different experimental animals. Then 4,000 healthy men were put on regular gossypol treatment for up to four years. Close on 100 per cent of them became infertile as judged by sperm counts of zero or well below the usually accepted levels for fertility. Side-effects were said to be mild and uncommon.

So far, so good. This 'Chinese sperm take-away', as it has been called, certainly seems a promising male contraceptive. However, there have been so many disappointments in this field of research into new methods for men, that we cannot be optimistic before far more exhaustive safety checks which are being done through the World Health Organization have been completed. Side-effects are proving more of a problem than was first suggested by the Chinese scientists. The chief one is a feeling of weakness, probably connected with a lowering of potassium in the body. Digestive disturbances and loss of sex drive are reported. And often there is such an extremely long recovery time necessary before the number and appearance of the sperm returns to normal, that doubts have been expressed about gossypol's reversibility at all in some men.

Animal research shows no effects on the hormones FSH and LH, which is good, but hamsters fail to put on weight normally when given gossypol. In summary it looks unlikely that gossypol itself will prove to be that elusive safe reversible male contraceptive. But the initial lead has been most helpful, and there is hope that variants produced by the chemists may result in a product suitable for use by ordinary couples.

Maturing of the sperm in the epididymis (stage ♂2)

The epididymis is a very long (7 metres), fine coiled-up tube, which forms into something about the size of a baby's little finger closely applied to the testicle. It receives the sperm leaving the production line in the testicle and its main job is to deliver at the other end, at the start of the vas, sperm which are now mature and able to swim. Several drugs have been found to interfere with this maturing process. The great advantage of acting at this stage, if only a safe drug could be discovered, is that there would be a far more rapid loss and return of fertility than by any of the methods above which interfere with sperm manufacture. The treatment should affect within a few days only those sperm which are just ready for ejaculation. And when the drug is stopped, once any (perhaps damaged) sperm have been flushed out, the ones arriving fresh from the production line should hopefully not have been affected by it.

One of the first drugs tested for this effect was called *alpha-chlorohydrin*. More recently, *derivatives of ordinary sugar,* modified and containing chlorine atoms, had seemed very promising. In animal experiments they interfered with the fertilizing ability of already manufactured sperm, and when the treatment was stopped the animals were fertile again within a week. None of the drugs so far discovered has been found to be safe enough to use in man as they are toxic to the bone marrow and nervous system. But the basic idea is sound, and non-toxic alternatives are being sought.

Another spin-off from this research is that these chemicals, and also gossypol derivatives, are showing promise as more effective vaginal spermicides than those at present available.

Sperm transport from the epididymis onwards (stage ♂3)

Transport through the vas (stage ♂3a)

Vasectomy deserves to be and is very popular. It is a minor operation, basically a 'plumbing-job'. A small section of the vas is removed and the ends closed with catgut or by cautery (heat).

There are no proven serious long-term unwanted effects in men. It is true that in both men and animals antibodies to sperm appear in quite a proportion. However, these are apparently not harmful in men; they do not even appear to interfere too much with the fertility of any individual after reversal of the operation. In spite of scare stories in the newspapers there is to date no hard evidence that these antibodies or any other effect of vasectomy can cause harm to the health of men after vasectomy. In this important respect men seem to be different from certain well-publicized monkeys studied in the USA.

217

Vasectomy taps?

Vasectomy can be reversed, even when the original procedure was done by the usual methods. Using the operating microscope a team from St Louis in the United States are claiming that 90 per cent of the men operated on achieved sperm counts in the normal range, although the highest pregnancy rate quoted is 70 per cent.

It is therefore attractive to consider devising some kind of *tap* which a man could turn on or off at will. Various such systems, one made of gold, have in fact been invented. They have not yet worked in practice because they were rejected by the tissues or became blocked. But even if taps were perfected, there is one snag which many people have not considered. Obviously turning the tap *on* should restore fertility almost at once. However, a man would have to wait perhaps up to three months after turning the tap off – just like after the original operation – before he could be sure that the downstream sperm had been flushed out and intercourse would not lead to a pregnancy. Ideally he should also get a pre-intercourse sperm count done. This is exactly the wrong way round, as many couples would happily wait three months to get their fertility back, but want their contraception to work straight away. This would not necessarily be a serious objection to the tap approach in a long-term relationship, however.

Transport through the male urethra (stage ♂3b)

The mythical intra-penile device would work at this point. So, obviously, does the sheath (condom). Research is going on into 'disappearing' soluble sheaths, which are made of a film of actual spermicide and are designed to dissolve during intercourse. Judging by past experience of spermicides used alone, this is unlikely to provide good protection against pregnancy.

Research is also going on, as in women, into *immune methods*. So far progress has been disappointing there as well.

The fact is that the practical male methods available now, or likely to appear in the near future, remain, apart from withdrawal, simply the sheath and vasectomy. This is regrettable as women would very reasonably like men to take their share in this matter of birth control, and many men would like to be able to do just that. As making love itself is very much a sharing business, we badly need an adequately safe pill for each sex – so that partners could take turns at being responsible for contraception. Each would then be exposed to half the long-term risks of the methods.

Conclusion

This chapter could do no more than give a general framework for understanding future advances in family planning, and there has only been space for a few examples. The main thing to remember is that any future method you hear about has to be based on detecting or interfering with one of the stages in Figure 19.

Secondly, if you read reports of new methods, always be sceptical. Far too little money and scientific attention is directed to contraceptive research. In many countries drug regulatory committees have been created. They aim to ensure that new medicines and techniques are as safe as can be. But in the contraceptive drug field their understandable caution has the effect of making development of new methods so expensive and prolonged (15 years is the minimum) as to tend to stop it altogether. Journalists often suggest that a brand-new method is just around the corner, when in fact it could be early next century before it is cleared for general use, if at all. This can be irritating to many who find all the available methods unsatisfactory for one reason or another.

Thirdly, many women feel that they were betrayed during the 1960s over the problems of the original combined pill. Doctors are accused, not always fairly, of doing too little to warn users that there could be long-term problems. It seemed at that time a magical method, a panacea, 'the pill of the Brave New World'. Time has shown up its drawbacks, but these too have often been exaggerated. These lessons must be learned and applied when any new pill comes along, whether for use by men or by women.

Yet, for obvious reasons, the best of any future methods which may be devised will be those which act at just one stage in the reproductive process, and do not have any effects on the whole body at all – except good ones perhaps!

10

All things considered: shall I take the pill?

The final decision has to be your own: books and doctors can only answer your questions, so far as the facts are known, and maybe give you some unbiased advice. But it is up to you to weigh up all the pros and cons, in consultation with your partner, and decide which method will suit you both best.

Your own 'best' method will depend on many things, among them: how crucial it is that you do not get pregnant; how much medical risk you feel prepared to accept; and how the actual method fits in with your sex life. Table 13 summarizes most of the pros and cons of the main recommended effective methods of birth control which are widely available, and may help you to make up your mind. Notice that injectables such as *Depo-Provera* are not shown here, because they are not widely available, though I believe they ought to be, as one of a couple's possible choices. See pages 202–3. The other methods which are *not* in the Table are missed out for the good reason that in the experience of most of the people who use them, they have a high failure rate. Notice particularly that no variety of *spermicide* is recommended for use on its own, even though in some countries various spermicides are heavily promoted by the manufacturers who imply that they are much more effective than they are. They appear in many different guises: pessaries, foaming tablets, creams, gels, ovals, films and foams. Of course they are a great deal better than nothing and the same applies to the *withdrawal method,* which some couples have used successfully for many years. But even if it works it does tend to be rather frustrating. So are the present ovulation or *'natural methods'*; but future

Table 13 The main recommended and widely available methods of birth control

A. Reversible methods

Advantages	Disadvantages

The ordinary combined pill

Advantages	Disadvantages
1. Extremely effective against pregnancy. Pregnancy rate in the range 0.1–1 per 100 woman-years	1. Medical supervision required.
	2. Needs a reasonably good memory to take the pills regularly.
	3. Minor problems such as weight gain (page 137).
2. Independent of intercourse	4. A slight chance of major problems such as thrombosis.
3. Beneficial effects, especially on the symptoms of the menstrual cycle. See page 137.	5. Especially unsuitable for women aged over 30–35 who are also heavy smokers.
	6. Some of the possible long-term consequences are still unknown.

The progestogen-only pill (mini-pill): see Chapter 8

Advantages	Disadvantages
1. Effective against pregnancy. Pregnancy rate 0.5–4 per 100 woman-years, the lower figure applying to older women.	1. Medical supervision required.
2. Independent of intercourse.	2. Needs to be taken obsessionally regularly.
3. Probably medically safer than the combined pill, as much less hormone is taken.	3. Minor problems, especially with the menstrual cycle.
4. Can be used by women aged over 40 and others for whom the combined pill is not recommended, or is proving unsatisfactory.	4. Very slight chance of major problems including ectopic pregnancy.
	5. Some of the possible long-term consequences still unknown.

IUD (loop or coil which is inserted into the uterus)

Advantages	Disadvantages
1. Effective against pregnancy. Pregnancy rate 0.5–4 per 100 woman-years, the lower figure applying to older women.	1. Medical supervision required.
2. Independent of intercourse.	2. At insertion: can cause discomfort, and there is a very slight chance of perforation of the uterus.
3. Nothing to remember: nothing to take or use daily.	3. The device may get expelled from the uterus into the vagina. This has to be watched out for.
4. No systemic effects, on the whole body.	4. May cause cramps, and heavy or prolonged or unpredictable bleeding.
5. Overall risk of death the same as or less than if the combined pill is used and, unlike it, becomes medically safer the older the user becomes.	5. Has certain medical risks, among them pelvic infection, miscarriage, and ectopic pregnancy. Pelvic infection is *rare, except* in IUD-users risking STD (page 20).

[*continued overleaf*]

Table 13 (*cont.*)

A. Reversible methods

Advantages	Disadvantages
	6. Because the problems mentioned at 5 can lead to damage to one or both of the uterine tubes and hence interfere with future fertility, *not* an ideal method for women who have not yet had their family. Particularly unsuitable for most women under the age of 20.

The sheath (preferably used with a spermicidal pessary, or lubricated with a spermicide)

1. Effective if used with care. Pregnancy rate can be as low as the IUD but very much depends on the user.	1. Needs very careful and consistent use.
2. Easy to obtain at odd hours.	2. Forward planning necessary, to have the sheath available every time.
3. Good for infrequent intercourse.	3. Not independent of intercourse. Seems a 'messy' intrusion into love-making for some.
4. May help a man who tends to climax too soon.	4. Both partners may be aware that it is being used. Loss of sensitivity is much less with the newest, thinner varieties which are spermicidally lubricated.
5. Visual proof that it has 'worked'.	5. Can slip off or rupture in use.
6. NO MEDICAL RISKS WHATEVER.	
7. No medical supervision required.	
8. Protects against picking up or passing on sexually transmitted diseases and perhaps cancer of the cervix in the woman (not completely protective though).	

The cap which *must* be used with a spermicide (e.g. the diaphragm, which is put in by the woman to cover the entrance to the uterus)

1. Effective if used with care. Pregnancy rate can be as low as the IUD but very much depends on the user.	1. Medical supervision required, to choose the right size of cap and to be trained to use it properly.
2. More independent of intercourse than the sheath. Can be put in as a routine ahead of time and should not therefore interfere with spontaneity.	2. Needs very careful and consistent use.
3. Neither partner usually notices any loss of sensitivity.	3. Forward planning necessary.
	4. Seems a bit messy to some.
4. If properly fitted and used, virtually no side-effects.	5. Diaphragm may increase the likelihood of bladder infections in some women. Other types of cap may be preferable if this is a problem.
5. Protects somewhat against sexually transmitted diseases, and perhaps cancer of the cervix.	

Table 13 (*cont.*)

B. Methods which are not readily reversible – sterilization in either sex

Advantages	Disadvantages

General pros and cons of sterilization in either sex

Advantages	Disadvantages
1. Almost 100 per cent effective.	1. Not readily reversible – but pregnancy rates after reversal operations by experts can be better than 50 per cent.
2. Independent of intercourse.	
3. Nothing to be taken daily.	2. An operation is required with more or less discomfort and inconvenience.
4. Medical supervision and possible problems only during the year of operation.	
5. No known long-term medical effects of importance, in the human.	

Pros and cons of female sterilization by blocking the uterine tubes

Advantages	Disadvantages
1. Once a woman decides to be sterilized, she is less likely in later years to want it reversed than a man might do, because nature will sterilize her anyway around the age of 50 (the menopause).	1. Medical risks of the operation are greater than vasectomy, though still small. Latest techniques using clips or rings are much safer than before.
2. The operation is immediately effective.	2. Usually requires admission to hospital and frequently a general anaesthetic.
	3. If the operation fails, which it can very rarely do in the early months, there is a risk of ectopic pregnancy.
	4. Psychologically, though illogically, women may feel no longer so feminine because they cannot have babies.

Pros and cons of vasectomy (male sterilization) by blocking the vas deferens

Advantages	Disadvantages
1. Almost completely safe medically.	1. Occasional short-term local complications of the operation, such as swellings or infection.
2. Can be done under local anaesthetic, as an out-patient, almost anywhere.	2. The operation takes three or more months to become effective.
3. There is a ready check of success by doing sperm counts.	3. Especially if they re-marry, more older men than women will wish for a reversal operation (see the point about the menopause, above).
4. It is more readily reversible than the female operation. With vasectomy reversal (like the original operation) there is no need for a surgeon to enter the abdomen. The reversal operation can also be repeated, if necessary.	4. Psychologically, though illogically, some men may feel 'threatened' by the operation, and may seem to overcompensate needlessly to show how manly they still are.
	5. Some *remotely* possible long-term effects still unknown, but all recent human evidence is reassuring (page 217).

developments may lead to more reliability with less abstaining necessary. See page 211.

An extra advantage of both the sheath and the cap is that they only need to be used when necessary. There is none of the feeling that some women get when taking pills, for instance, that it all seems rather pointless a lot of the time because intercourse is infrequent or unpredictable.

A note about the so-called 'messiness' of barrier methods of family planning such as *the sheath and the cap*. I am sure this has been much exaggerated. And even if partly true, it is worth pondering the following comment which was made by a woman journalist: ' . . . But women's lives are messy; it is messy to bleed once a month; it is messy to give birth; sex itself is not for the fastidious.'

How to plan your family planning

Some people will use only one or two methods of family planning throughout their lives; others will 'ring the changes' between the various methods shown in Table 13; for some a method such as the pill may be out of the question because of a medical contra-indication. But one thing is clear: whatever else applies, the best choice of method is likely to vary with time, or according to what I call in Table 14 'The seven contraceptive ages of woman'. But I do emphasize that Table 14 is just a guide: the choice of method of contraception is a very individual thing and no one method is ever ideal and best for everyone, even within a particular one of the seven categories. Not all the satisfactory options are even mentioned. The scheme only represents the 'state of the art' based on the methods available at the start of the 1980s. If some of the ideas in Chapter 9 become practical possibilities for ordinary couples to use, then the ideal system might very well change.

Table 14 represents an ideal scheme, so it is assumed that the woman concerned will be a non-smoker and will, if she can, breast-feed her children. It is also assumed that she or her partner will use whatever method is chosen responsibly and consistently.

A main point to notice in the Table is that the pill is often the ideal method early on in fertile life, and if used at all the other

224

Table 14 The seven contraceptive ages of woman

'Age'	Suggested method
1. Birth to puberty:	No method required. However, responsible matter-of-fact sex education is essential – principally from the parents.
2. Puberty to marriage:	Either (a) a barrier method (*sheath* or *cap* plus spermicide) or (b) *the combined pill*, or (c) the 'best' oral contraceptive (i.e. saying 'no'). Choice depends on factors like religious views, the steadiness of the relationship, and frequency of intercourse.
3. Marriage to first child:	First choice usually the *combined pill*, followed by a *barrier method* for three months before 'trying' for the first child (pp.63–4).
4. During breast-feeding:	First choice: *barrier method* (perhaps taking it in turns to use either the *cap* or the *sheath*). Second choice: (a) *IUD* (but a small risk to future fertility), (b) *progestogen-only pill* (but unknown effect of the minute amount of hormone transferred in the breast milk).
5. Family spacing after breast-feeding:	Continue with method started during 4, or shift to *combined pill* at this time for greater effectiveness and a regular bleeding pattern.
6. After the (probable) last child:	First choice: *IUD*. Other possibles: *barrier methods* or the *progestogen-only pill*, according to choice.
7. Family complete, children growing up and other methods unacceptable:	*Vasectomy*; or *female sterilization* using clips or rings.

main reversible medical method of family planning, the IUD, is best reserved until later. This is because the known medical risks of the pill are less when you are young, and the younger you are the more secure you usually want to be against pregnancy. Besides, the 'fringe-benefits' like shorter and less painful periods are particularly appreciated. On the other hand, the coil is relatively bad news for young women who have not yet completed their families, as it can cause various complications which could prejudice the chance of having a baby later. These are pelvic infection (infection of the uterine tubes); ectopic pregnancy; unplanned pregnancy in the uterus, often in that case leading to miscarriage which can, rarely, be followed by infection in the tubes. However, by the sixth age in the Table, when your family is probably complete, but you are not yet quite ready for sterilization, those worries about the IUD are much less important. In addition most of the problems of the coil are less frequent in older women anyway. Moreover, unplanned pregnancy due to the device failing is definitely less likely in older women. So the coil really comes into its own at the very time it is likely to be needed as an alternative because the risks of the pill are definitely increased in older women. The IUD can be a very useful 'holding manoeuvre' before your husband has his vasectomy (or you your sterilization).

Sterilization of either partner is often the ideal once the family is complete, because it is so safe medically and so effective against unplanned 'afterthoughts'. If you do not smoke, often it may be reasonable to take the slightly increasing medical risks with age of staying on the combined pill right through until either you or your partner is sterilized. However, it is not intended to imply that *everyone* should finish up by being sterilized. Indeed, it is important to remember about *female* sterilization that its risks become relatively more important after a woman reaches 40, because there are then fewer years left in which to get the benefit from it before she reaches the menopause. Of course, how long this will be cannot be estimated in advance at all accurately. All that can be done is to balance the likely number of years of protection provided by the sterilization against the risks that are run during the actual year the operation is done. In developed countries the average age of the menopause is about 50.

Apart from sterilization, what methods are suitable for people during the seventh age, from the time when they are sure that their family is complete through until the time of the menopause? By the time they reach their forties a sizeable minority of around 10 per cent of women in Britain, and up to three times that number in some countries, have had their uterus removed (hysterectomy) for problems such as very heavy bleeding. Hysterectomy is of course a method of sterilization. Like the more usual method of blocking the uterine tubes, once the operation has been successfully performed it has no known long-term medical side-effects whatsoever (provided at least one ovary is left behind). But it is too big a procedure to be done routinely for family planning purposes. When it is medically indicated, good counselling is vital, as for other forms of sterilization.

In fact, many couples manage perfectly well using reversible methods of family planning right through to the menopause. Many women find the IUD or the progestogen-only pill entirely satisfactory (but see page 195). Such women do, however, have to bear in mind that if they get irregular bleeding they should see their doctor to be sure it does not have a gynaecological explanation, before they assume it is due to their method. A surprisingly large number of people simply use the sheath or the cap at this time. Whatever reversible method is used, it should not normally be abandoned until one year after the very last menstrual period, as pregnancy during this time is not entirely unknown following an unexpected delayed egg-release. (But a blood test may be helpful – see page 195).

Combinations of methods

Some people really have difficulty in finding any method at all that suits them. Contraception can then be the source of a lot of tension and frustration. Occasionally a workable solution may be found if the partners, so to speak, share the contraceptive load: for instance, sometimes using the sheath and sometimes the diaphragm plus spermicide. Or a woman who feels motivated enough to persevere with the temperature method may use that to identify the only genuinely safe time – from three days after the temperature goes up after egg-release through until the start of the next period – while her partner uses a method like the sheath, which they may not much care for, during the rest of the menstrual cycle.

Using combinations of methods in a different way can help people who are terrified that a method will let them down. For example, the IUD can fail: especially in younger women under 30. If, however, they make a point of inserting a spermicidal pessary regularly every time before love-making, the effectiveness of their method can be improved.

Conclusion

Looking back over this chapter, and over the whole book, it is impossible to avoid one conclusion. A lot of the time in family planning we, and for the most part unfortunately that means women, are having to 'make the best of a bad job'. While we can hope for a successful outcome to some of the research described in Chapter 9, we have to *lead our sex lives now, with the methods actually available now*.

If you do decide to take the pill, and currently this is the most effective reversible method, make sure it is an informed decision which seems right to you and is not influenced by pressure from anyone else: your partner, the media, let alone any doctor. If you decide the pill is not for you, be sure to use some reliable alternative. Sex and birth control are matters which affect your body; they are your responsibility and require your decisions. That sums up the purpose for which this book was written.

100 questions everyone asks about the pill

Introduction

The answers to the questions here are deliberately very brief and hence sometimes over-simplified. Please refer to the pages mentioned for more details.

The two main types of pill are: POP = progestogen-only pill, OCP = ordinary combined pill. As in the rest of this book, the OCP is often just called the pill, and because it is much more widely used than the POP, most of the questions and answers below refer to it.

(a) Types of pill and how they work

1. *What is the ordinary combined pill (OCP)?*
   This contains an oestrogen and progestogen and is usually taken daily, for 21 days out of every 28.

2. *How does it work?*
   Chiefly by stopping maturing and release of eggs (Chapter 2).

3. *What is the mini-pill/progestogen-only pill (POP)?*
   As its name suggests, this contains only a progestogen in very low dose, and is taken every single day of the year without breaks (Chapter 8).

4. *How does the POP work?*
   Chiefly by altering the cervical mucus to stop sperm entering the uterus, and by various changes to the lining of the uterus. See Chapter 8 for more details about this and other aspects of the POP.

5. *How effective are pills against pregnancy?*
   Very, if regularly taken. The failure rate of the OCP is 0.1 to 1.0 pregnancies per hundred woman-years (page 38). The figure for the POP is 0.5 to 4 per hundred woman-years (page 183).

6. *Are all the combined pills the same?*
No, there are differences between the brands, but we do not know which is the 'best buy' (pages 131–3). It seems best to take the lowest possible dose of both hormones: hence ultra-low-dose pills and POPs (Table 11, page 194) are preferred. But every woman is different, and some need the slightly higher-dose pills of Table 9 (page 163).

7. *What about phased pills?*
These are OCPs giving a daily dose of both progestogen and oestrogen, but the ratio of one hormone to the other varies stepwise (see page 168 for details). They may be either biphasic (two phases) or triphasic (three phases). Their main advantage is that they usually give a good pattern of bleeding. Those available in Britain are ultra-low dose, but this is not necessarily true everywhere (see pages 266–70).

8. *How long has the pill been available?*
The initial trials were in America and Puerto Rico in 1956. It was first marketed in the US in 1960, reaching most other countries in the early 1960s.

(b) Availability of the pill

9. *How can I get a supply of the pill?*
In Britain over 90 per cent of family doctors will prescribe the pill. If your doctor will not, you should be able to obtain it from another local doctor, even if he or she is in a different practice; or from a Family Planning Clinic (addresses in the telephone directory).

10. *But I am under the age of consent . . . Will they insist on telling my parents?*
These questions are answered on pages 67–8.
If question 10 applies to you, the short sections on Responsibility (pages 21–3) and Sexually Transmitted Diseases (pages 19–21) might also be worth reading.

11. *Can my partner come to the clinic or surgery with me?*
Certainly and, if you ask, he can usually also come in with you when you see the doctor.

12. *Do I have to be examined internally at the first visit?*

No. The internal examination is primarily to do with preventive medicine. See pages 66–7. Once you are a pill-taker, regular checks of blood pressure and of headache pattern, breast examinations, and cervical smears are important (page 160).

13. *How often should I have a smear test done?*
This depends: policy varies from one district to another, so follow the advice of your doctor. An important factor is your own life-style (page 21), which could mean the need for annual testing whatever the local policy.

14. *They have asked me to come back for a smear test in only three months: what does this mean? Can I continue on the pill?*
No reason to panic: all this means is that a few abnormal cells have been found in the previous smear. Quite often these are got rid of by the body without any further treatment, and so are not seen on the repeat smear. Otherwise the doctor will discuss the whole matter with you. He or she will explain that even persistent changes in the smear can be readily dealt with and actual cancer of the cervix – which in any case would not occur for many years – can be prevented altogether by minor treatment, usually as an out-patient. See pages 21 and 67. And you should continue on the pill at least until you see your doctor, and possibly much longer – discuss in the light of pages 122, 153.

15. *How often should I attend the clinic or surgery for my pills?*
This will usually be determined by the number of packets you are given at each visit. Commonly you will be seen three months after first starting on the pill, and then regularly every six months. However, you must feel free to come back sooner than your next routine visit if you ever have any anxiety about using the pill or about any effect it seems to be having on you. See also Question 20 below about special medical supervision.

(c) Practical pill-taking

16. *Which diseases that I have ever suffered from should I be sure to mention to the doctor?*

231

The main thing to mention is any past thrombosis or any disease or disorder affecting the circulation (pages 149–51). These include diabetes, high blood pressure, and heavy cigarette-smoking. Liver troubles should be mentioned; the other important short- and long-term disorders are to be found on pages 149–60. Allergies, especially to drugs, should also be entered in your case notes.

17. *What diseases in my family are important?*

Once again, any history of thrombosis or any kind of stroke is important, but only if it affected a near-relative at a young age (say under 50). Mention also if there is a family tendency to breast cancer, or raised blood pressure or diabetes (page 156). When in doubt mention any unusual family complaint, especially porphyria (page 152) and otosclerosis (page 154).

18. *Who should never take the pill?*

Having noted the diseases in your own past or still affecting you, or those which run in your family, the final decision about this will be taken by your doctor in consultation with you. See pages 149–55.

19. *Who should be very cautious about taking the pill and then only with special medical supervision?*

Again, this will depend on your own medical history and that of your family (pages 155–60). If one of these 'relative contra-indications' applies, it is usually essential to use an OCP giving the minimum possible dose – or the POP (page 194).

20. *What does 'special medical supervision' mean?*

It means (page 160) being seen by the doctor more often than usual, being told what to look out for so as to return earlier if necessary, and sometimes having special tests done. It also means being ready to discontinue the pill should some condition worsen, or a new risk factor or problem appear.

21. *There seems to be no medical objection, so how do I start taking the pill?*

There are two main ways of starting the OCP, on day five or on day one of the period (pages 43–6 and Figures 9 and 10). The POP should always be started on day one (page

184). See also pages 46, 184 for how to start OCPs and POPs after any kind of recent pregnancy.

22. *Which pill is best if I plan to breast-feed my baby?*
The POP – but first read carefully the discussion on page 196.

23. *How soon after starting the pill am I protected against pregnancy?*
At once, if either OCP or POP are started early enough after a full-term baby; or if the OCP is started by the day after a miscarriage or termination of pregnancy, or on day one of the menstrual cycle. In *all* other circumstances – except perhaps when starting POP directly after the OCP – alternative precautions such as the sheath should be used until 14 tablets have been taken (pages 43–6, 184).

24. *How do I take the pills after that?*
You take 21 consecutive daily pills followed by a 7-day break for all the OCPs except Minilyn (page 163). Every Day pills contain dummies to be taken during the pill-free week. Like them, the POP is taken every single day including during periods. With *all* pills tablet-taking should continue following the daily routine, even if there is unexpected bleeding (pages 60 and 183 and Question 51 below).

25. *Is it safe to make love on the days when OCPs are not taken?*
Yes: *but only* if no pills have been missed (or not absorbed) towards the end of the previous pill packet, and you do in fact start another packet after the pill-free week (page 43).

26. *Do I have to take pills at the same time of day, and if so what time is best?*
For OCPs, any regular time will do. POPs should be taken within an hour of the same time each day. For many the best time is in the early evening. The worst time for this pill is just before the usual time for love-making (page 184).

27. *How can I ever remember to take my pills?*
Some women find it helpful to take one of the Every Day packs of OCPs, which contain 21 active tablets and

233

7 dummies so there is no need to remember when to stop and start successive courses. Get your pill-taking routine linked with something else that you do regularly every day. For instance, you could tie your packet of OCPs to your tooth-brush. An alarm watch set to 7 o'clock in the evening may be safest for the POP.

28. *I have forgotten to take a pill: am I certain to get pregnant?*
No, especially if you are on the OCP, and with both types of pill if you do not rely on pills for the recommended time (see Question 29).

29. *What shall I do?*
OCPs: if more than 12 hours late in pill-taking, take the missing pill(s) and then continue in all respects as usual with your pill-taking routine, but use the sheath or a similar method for the next 14 days (see Figure 11 and pages 49–51 for further details). The rules for the POP are similar but the 14-day rule must be followed if only 3 hours late in taking a tablet (see Figure 18, pages 188–9, and the Important Note on page 185).

30. *What shall I do if I have a stomach upset – vomiting or diarrhoea?*
As far as your body is concerned, this can be like missing a tablet. See Figures 12 or 18 (pages 54–5, 188–9) for the rules to be followed with OCPs or POPs for maximum peace of mind.

31. *Can other medicines affect the reliability of the OCPs and POPs?*
Yes, some can. This particularly applies to some antibiotics and to treatments for tuberculosis and for epilepsy. Bleeding on OCP-taking days may be an early warning sign (Table 2a and pages 56–8,186).

32. *Can the pill affect the actions of other medicines?*
Again, this is possible, depending on the nature of the other treatment. See Table 2b and page 58, for OCPs: there are no reports of this with POPs.

33. *Should I then always make a special point of telling any doctor who sees me that I am on the pill?*
Yes. This is vital, not only because of this problem of interaction between drugs, but also because laboratory

tests may be affected (page 74); and the knowledge that you are on OCP or POP may also help when making a diagnosis.

34. *Does it matter if I accidentally take more than one pill per day?*

No. In fact this is sometimes recommended (Figure 11, page 50). However, if you make this mistake, it is best to take your *next* pill from another packet, so that the day of pill-taking matches the day marked on your packet.

35. *If a change to a different brand of OCP is recommended, are there any special rules?*

Yes. If moving to a pill on the same 'rung' of Figure 15 (pages 165–7), or higher, just take the usual 7-day break between old and new packets. But if moving *down* to a lower-dose pill, take the first new packet without any break after the old one (page 59). See page 168 for the rules for phased pills, and page 185 if moving to POP, or from POP to any other method.

36. *If I lose my OCPs half-way through a packet and my friend has a spare packet of a different brand, is it safe to take them?*

Forget this if either yours or hers are phased pills (page 168). Even if they are of the fixed-dose type, it is *not* recommended. However, if there seems no alternative, perhaps when you are away for a weekend, then you should certainly check that the pill is on an equivalent rung of the ladders of Figure 15. If it is higher, protection will be maintained, but if lower, then it may be reduced and you should preferably follow the 14-day loss-of-protection rule, as well as taking the new pills. (The same rule, or that on page 59, is best followed when you return to your normal pill from a borrowed higher-dose one!)

37. *What shall I do if I need some more pills when in a foreign country?*

Look up your variety of pill in the World directory of pill names (page 266). You should then be able to use the name of the nearest equivalent locally available brand when you visit the doctor or chemist.

38. *If my partner goes abroad, or I get a side-effect, can I stop the pill in the middle of a packet?*

With the OCP it is best to complete the packet. But if you have one of the possibly serious symptoms mentioned on pages 61–2, you should still be able to avoid a pregnancy if you transfer immediately to using another method like the sheath. POPs are best stopped during a period (page 185) so this could be before the end of a packet.

39. *Does it matter if I take the pill for short spells of a few months at a time, according to need?*
No, so long as the rules for starting and stopping are followed each time (see Questions 23, 25 and 38).

40. *If I want a baby, can I just stop the pill? Or should I use another method for a while?*
See page 110 for the answer to this one and to Question 77 (about pill-taking *during* pregnancy). It seems that previous use of the pill does not increase the chance of having an abnormal baby, though the evidence is conflicting.

41. *What should I do if I am not quite sure whether I have had German measles? Or whether I was vaccinated against it as a schoolgirl?*
German measles in early pregnancy can harm babies, so you should not stop the pill until you have had the blood test to check that you are immune (page 68).

42. *If I am not immune, how long must I wait after the vaccination for German measles before getting pregnant?*
Three months (page 69). So it is logical to get this matter sorted out while you are still taking the OCP or POP, or using some other effective method.

43. *I am going into hospital for an operation – should I stop the pill and if so, when? And when can I take it again?*
Much depends on whether this is for a major or a minor operation. If you are told you will be in hospital for a week or more after the operation, then you should transfer from the OCP to another effective method six weeks beforehand. There is normally no need to discontinue the POP in this way, but discuss the matter with your doctor. If there are no complications you can restart the pill *at the first subsequent period which comes on at least four weeks after the operation.*

44. *Does being sterilized count as a major operation?*
These days, usually not: as by modern techniques you can usually go home within a day or two. Therefore there is no need to stop the OCP, and usually it is best to continue pill-taking after the operation until the end of the current packet.

45. *How long can I stay on the pill? Should I make a break every two years? Or after five years?*
The effect of the length of pill-use on the risks of diseases of the circulation and cancer has not yet been fully worked out (pages 126–30). But it is clear that the uncommon infertility problem of amenorrhoea – absent periods for many months – after stopping the pill is no more likely after long-term than short-term use. So it is not necessary, as used to be recommended, to make a routine break every two years.

According to present knowledge and depending on other factors which apply to you, it is preferable after about ten years' use of the OCP *to begin to consider whether to move to another method.* However it could be OK for you to use it for longer, especially if you are a non-smoker (pages 126–30, 157–8). (Even less is known about the risks, if any, of long-term use of the POP – though they are thought to be less than those of the OCP.)

(d) Pills and periods, or no periods

• Ordinary combined pill (OCP)

46. *What causes 'periods' on the OCP? Are they really periods at all?*
The natural menstrual cycle is abolished whether or not you see any bleeding. It is replaced by the pill cycle in which bleeding is caused in a quite different way, by withdrawal of the hormones from the blood supply to the uterus for 7 days out of every 28. So they are not true periods (page 38 and Figure 8).

47. *I have irregular periods naturally – can I take the pill?*
This depends: special tests may be required. An important factor is whether you would accept an alternative (not the IUD). See pages 109 and 158.

48. *I have missed a 'period' – what shall I do?*

If you have no reason to suspect loss of protection by the pill (pages 49–59), you should start a new packet after the pill-free week in the usual way. However, if the next pill withdrawal bleed also fails to come – i.e. you miss two 'periods' in a row – you should see your doctor before starting another packet (page 53).

49. *If I don't see much of a 'period' on the pill/I see no bleeding at all in the pill-free week, is blood collecting inside me?*

No – as explained on pages 38–40, if you have no bleeding it simply means there is no blood to come away. Check you are not pregnant, and then if you wish you can continue with the pill (Figure 17b, pages 175–7), if your doctor agrees.

50. *Can I avoid having monthly bleeding altogether – e.g. when going on holiday?*

Yes: the best way is to take two packets in a row (page 43). But there are special rules for phased pills (page 169).

51. *What is the tricycle pill?*

This is the ordinary pill, but refers to a system of taking four packets in a row followed by a 7-day break (page 42). It gives only four hormone withdrawal bleeds a year, but does mean that over all more hormone is taken in the time. NB Do not confuse this with the triphasic pill – see Question 7.

52. *I am bleeding like a period on days of pill-taking: should I stop in the middle of a packet?*

On no account! The golden rule of pill-taking is to carry on taking your pills according to the 21 days on, 7 days off routine, irrespective of the pattern of bleeding or no-bleeding which may occur. See page 174 (Figure 17a) and make an early appointment to discuss this with your doctor, particularly if it is a new problem.

53. *I not only get spotting on pill-taking days, I have had no bleeding during the last seven days of no tablet-taking! What shall I do?*

Actually, this is quite a common combination of problems. If you have no reason to suspect loss of protection from the pill, and this is the first missed 'period', then follow the rules at Question 48 above and start taking your next packet on the correct day. If you persevere, taking your pills regularly, there is a good chance that the correct bleeding pattern will be established. If not, you should make an early appointment to discuss things with your doctor (Figure 17 and pages 174–7).

Irregular bleeding like this is even more likely to happen after erratic pill-taking, or some other reason for loss of protection (pages 49–59). If this applies to you, then follow the rules of Figures 11 or 12 and page 53, and take your doctor's advice before starting another packet.

● *Progestogen-only pill (POP)*

54. *What causes periods on the POP?*
Quite unlike the OCP, these periods are natural ones: due to the loss of the natural progesterone and oestrogen, as egg-release and formation of a corpus luteum usually occur (page 182).

55. *Does it matter if I see no periods on the POP?*
Yes and no. First check you are not pregnant. If not, this means you are as protected against pregnancy as if you were on the OCP (page 187). It may mean your natural menstrual cycle is particularly easy to stop; the POP should not be appreciably harming your fertility and can be continued. See page 190 and discuss the matter with your doctor.

56. *What should I do if I get erratic bleeding and spotting on the POP?*
Continue daily pill-taking: if the bleeding pattern is unacceptable see your doctor.

● *Periods after stopping the pill – either OCP or POP.*

57. *Although I had very regular 'periods' on the pill I stopped it some months ago and have seen no periods yet. What does this mean?*
It means that your natural menstrual cycle, with egg-release and periods, has not been restored. It usually will be without treatment (pages 63, 109 and see Question 58).

239

58. *We have been trying to have a baby since stopping the pill with no success yet. Was the pill to blame and should we have tests done?*

Ten to fifteen per cent of all couples have difficulty achieving a pregnancy, so it *could* be a coincidence. Discuss referral for tests with your doctor if you see no periods for six months or more, or you could wait a few months longer if periods have returned.

59. *Could using the pill for a long time make my menopause happen earlier? or later?*

Neither the OCP nor POP are thought to have any effect on the time of the menopause.

60. *If I am on the POP, how do I find out that I have reached the menopause?*

(No one should be on the OCP at this age of course.) The usual way is to transfer to another method. It may sometimes be possible to confirm the menopause by a blood test – discuss with your doctor and see page 195, also Question 76 below.

(e) Problems with the pill

61. *How dangerous, really, is the OCP?*

Like any drug it has risks, but these have often been exaggerated. One very good point is that no harm is likely to be caused by a large overdose (page 70).

62. *How dangerous is the POP?*

Probably even less so than the OCP (page 190).

63. *What side-effects will I notice?*

Often none at all. If you do, it is nearly always worth persevering (but see Question 64), at least for three months. Even then, do not give up the method too easily: as there are other brands of OCP or POP which might be tried.

64. *What symptoms should make me see a doctor at once?*

These are listed on pages 61–2, but they are very rare so do not let the list worry you!

65. *Won't I put on a lot of weight?*

Usually none with the POP, and very little if any with the

modern ultra-low-dose OCPs. But you may need to count calories a little more carefully (page 76). If you are already overweight, see pages 150, 158.

66. *Could the pill be causing my headaches?*
This is possible, especially on the pill-free days. Bad headaches or migraines should always be discussed with your doctor (pages 96–7).

67. *I get so depressed these days: how likely is it that the pill is to blame?*
There may sometimes be a clear-cut link with the pill (page 93).

68. *I seem to have lost interest in sex too; would stopping the pill help?*
Not very often. Transferring to an ultra-low-dose or oestrogen-dominant pill or the POP is worth trying first. If the problem is partly due to vaginal dryness, a jelly lubricant may also help (page 95).

69. *Could the brown blotches I have started to get on my face be due to the pill?*
Yes they could, they are given the name chloasma (p.115). The POP may help, if you still want to take a pill.

70. *Since starting on the pill I feel sick and dizzy and have too much vaginal discharge – what shall I do?*
All these may well improve after two or three courses of pills; nausea can often be reduced by taking the pills last thing at night. Otherwise these and other symptoms, which seem to be due to too much oestrogen effect in comparison with the progestogen effect, can be helped by using a progestogen-dominant pill, or by the progestogen-only pill (page 178).

71. *Thrombosis sounds very worrying: I am told it means clots, so does it mean that I can't use the pill if I have clots with my periods?*
Far from it: clots with the periods just mean that they are heavy, and could well improve dramatically if you went on the pill (page 107).

72. *What are the facts about thrombosis and other troubles of the circulation?*
Chapters 4 and 6 are mainly about this. In brief, the risk is

primarily in people who have other risk factors, listed on page 81. Smoking is the most common and main one, and becomes even more important as age increases (Table 4, page 90).

73. *Which reduces the risk more, to stop the pill or to stop smoking?*
This depends on how much you smoke, and other factors like which pill you take. For anyone smoking fifteen or more cigarettes a day, the risks of all the currently available pills are less over all than those of smoking. However long you have been a smoker, your chances of survival are always greater if you stop (page 91).

74. *I smoke twenty-five cigarettes a day: how can I be helped to stop?*
In Britain, ASH (Action on Smoking and Health – see useful addresses page 263) can give you practical advice, and there may be an anti-smoking clinic you could attend. But there is no magic method: you will never succeed unless you really want to give up, and are prepared to work hard to do so.

75. *At what age should I stop the pill?*
There is no set age. The risk increases steadily with time; it depends on whether you have any other risk factors, and is thought not to apply much to the POP. See Table 4, pages 89–92, 126–30, 157–8, 194, and discuss with your doctor.

76. *I am near the 'change of life', and I have been given treatment for hot flushes. The pills are in a packet which looks very like 'the Pill' and I take them just the same way. Are they contraceptives?*
No! If you were still having periods up to the time of starting this treatment, which is known as 'hormone replacement therapy', you should not rely on it. The dose system is different, and may not be effective in preventing pregnancy. See page 195.

77. *If I got pregnant and did not realize, would continuing to take the pill harm the baby?*
The risk of this is very low indeed, if it exists, and did not show up among 168 babies (page 110).

78. *Does the evidence we have so far suggest that the overall risk of cancer is greater in pill-users than those who never take the pill?*
No: see pages 119–24.

79. *Have the risks of the pill sometimes been exaggerated?*
Yes. Even more commonly, the problems of the pill are not put in perspective against its benefits, or in comparison with the risks and problems of alternatives, of using no method at all, and of life generally (pages 140–8).

80. *What about the risks for people in developing countries?*
These are probably less than in 'over-developed' countries, also the risks of alternatives and of pregnancy tend to be greater there. But much more research is needed (page 125).

81. *Are there still things we don't know about the pill, particularly about long-term risks?*
Yes (pages 126–30). This book can do no more than give a consensus or majority view on the known facts about the pill. Very preliminary findings are not mentioned, because it would be as wrong to cause false fears as it would be to raise false hopes.

82. *After all that, what good effects does the pill have?*
See Table 7 (pages 136–7). Main ones are that it is highly effective, acceptable, and unrelated to intercourse, and almost 100 per cent reversible; plus its good effects on the menstrual cycle in most women.

(f) People in special categories (if your situation is not mentioned here, please use the index)

83. *Does it affect my choice of pill that I am very underweight?*
Underweight women are more likely to have side-effects like menstrual cramps, nausea, and breast discomfort, and to have a long delay in return of their periods after stopping the pill. Hence they should be given either a combined pill with the lowest possible dose, or the POP (page 172).

84. *Can I take the combined pill if I have varicose veins?*
Yes, on their own these rarely mean that you must avoid the method. Please make a point of reading page 80.

85. *Can I take the pill if I am a diabetic?*
    Sometimes, but only with special medical supervision and for the shortest possible time (pages 150, 156).

86. *I am very troubled by acne, does this affect which pill I should take?*
    Yes it does: you should use a relatively oestrogen-dominant pill (pages 178–9).

87. *Can I use contact lenses if I take the pill?*
    Probably: with modern lenses and modern ultra-low-dose OCPs (and POPs). But if your eyes ever become sore do not use the lenses until you have seen your optician again for them to be examined, and for advice (page 98).

88. *I tend to be anaemic, can I take the pill?*
    It depends. If you have one of the commonest kinds of anaemia, due to heavy periods, the pill will be a great help (page 107). But if you have sickle cell anaemia (only possible if you have some negro blood in you) discuss the matter with your doctor (page 151).

89. *Does the fact that I have recently had infectious hepatitis (jaundice) mean that I cannot ever again take the pill?*
    No, but it does mean that you must have blood tests done to check when your liver is functioning normally, and you will usually be advised to stay off both OCP and POP for as long as you must avoid alcohol, normally about six months (page 152).

90. *What about the very itchy mild jaundice that I had in pregnancy?*
    This, like other conditions which are definitely or probably affected by any type of sex hormones (page 154), means you should always avoid the pill.

91. *Does it matter that I had high blood pressure (toxaemia) in pregnancy?*
    This must be mentioned to your doctor, and your blood pressure will need to be checked more often than usual. But most women with this history do not have any trouble later if they take the OCP (pages 82, 157).

92. *I had a funny kind of miscarriage, and am now having regular blood tests. What can this mean?*
    You presumably had a hydatidiform mole – ask your

doctor, and see page 123 for a full explanation. If so, you will have to avoid both the OCP and POP, but only till you are given the 'all-clear' by your doctor, based on the hCG tests.

(g) Miscellaneous

93. *Should I avoid any foods or alcohol, or take extra vitamins while on the pill?*
As a rule, no (pages 75–6). But see also pages 93–4, 111.

94. *What shall I do, my three-year-old daughter has just swallowed all the pills in my next packet . . . ?*
Nothing – provided you are sure that this is all she took. She may vomit, and within the next day or two she may have some painless bleeding from her uterus, like a light period. This sounds alarming but is actually no cause for concern (page 71).

95. *If the pill stops release of eggs, what happens to the eggs?*
They stay in the ovary, just as they would in a woman who was perpetually pregnant. However, there is always a steady loss of egg cells within the ovary, from before birth right through to the menopause (page 26).

96. *What is the injection/jab/jag/shot?*
These words and others are used to describe the injectable contraceptive called Depo-Provera, and various other progestogens which are being tried by this route (page 202).

97. *What is the 'morning-after' pill?*
This describes methods which are used after intercourse to prevent pregnancy. A lot of research is being done, but the few methods available now are only suitable for 'emergency' use. See pages 64, 205.

98. *What are 'once-a-month' pills?*
These are designed to cause the period to come on whether or not fertilization (and implantation) took place earlier that month. They are all research methods, apart from prostaglandins which can be used this way (page 205).

99. *What about the male pill?*
    I am sorry to say this is still very much in the future. There is no safe, acceptable pill for men now, nor is there likely to be one for several years to come (pages 212–19).

100. *What if I have any other questions about* ANYTHING?
    Ask them and keep on asking them: pertinent or impertinent questions! It is your body, you have a right to know. Never hesitate to go back to whoever prescribed your pills to discuss all aspects of pill-taking. But remember that some facts simply are not yet available.

Postscript

As I said on page 22, I feel no doctor involved in family planning should push his or her own moral views on those who come for advice. They should be met on their own ground. In all but the most unusual case, if an unmarried couple are having intercourse frequently it would be alienating and probably quite useless to suggest that they abstain. Circumstances vary, but the main thing is to help people avoid the nightmare of an unwanted pregnancy. I feel it is not my role to judge, but to care. Although my own views often differ from those to whom I prescribe the pill, to draw attention to this, except at their request, might mean losing the opportunity to help them (often not just with their contraception).

So I do prescribe the pill without moralizing to unmarried people: and also, with counselling, which is not the same as moralizing, to young teenagers. We live in the real world of the 1980s and my medical practice must be relevant to that world.

Though I must practise my profession in the real world this does not mean that I think all is well there in matters of sex and responsibility. Far from it. I am not in favour of the life-style that contributes to increasing numbers of broken marriages; single-parent families; induced abortions; not to mention prescriptions for tranquillizers for more and more insecure housewives and their partners, quite unable to trust each other. The 'copulation explosion' is the root cause of the epidemic of sexually transmitted diseases; and also, we now know, of abnormal cervical smears and the risk of cancer of the cervix. So I see it as sound medicine, not being 'holier than thou', to point out to a patient I have had to treat for pelvic infection due to a sexually transmitted disease that her future fertility could be damaged if she does not change her life-style; or to reinforce a teenager's wish, if she has it, *not* to be given the pill just yet, because she really does not feel ready for intercourse (or wishes to wait till she marries). Unfortunately, we live in a society which has rejected old values but can offer nothing satisfactory instead; a society where many young people receive little guidance, and plenty of bad examples. The pressures on them from the media and their friends are enormous, to the extent that it really seems to be abnormal not to be having sex at 16. Or, as a family doctor said, 'Sex at sixteen may be legal but it is not yet compulsory!'

Concerned as they rightly are to prevent unplanned pregnancy, sometimes school teachers and doctors can be implicated in these social pressures. They can find that their promotion of family planning is being seen as implying an official seal of approval for teenage sex.

The young will laugh at an arbitrary 'not at all', but will at least listen to a case for 'not yet', if it is factual and not linked to taboos or a negative attitude to sex. They need to know that the price to be paid for sexual intercourse in their early teens *can* be too high. At risk are self-respect, respect for others, and emotional security: their own and that of their children in the future. These facts apply to boys as well as girls. The sexual 'double standard' is offensive and must be abolished! But for girls there are also relevant medical facts: all contraceptives *can* fail, and the possible long-term risks may include infertility and even cancer (see pages 20 and 21).

The stakes are also high for adults. In the book *I Married You* (Further reading, page 258), the author compares sexual love to glue between two pieces of paper. 'If you try to separate two pieces of paper which are glued together, you tear them both. If you try to separate husband and wife who cleave together, both are hurt – and in those cases where they have children, the children as well. Divorce means to take a saw and to saw apart each child, from head to toe, right through the middle.' The imagery is too vivid, perhaps, but it rings true.

Personally, I am now a convinced Christian. I believe that the sexual behaviour we were designed for can be summed up as 'A one-man woman who makes love only with her one-woman man . . . for life'. I can accept that some who consider this notion old fashioned, and reject it, are nevertheless responsible. They can perhaps avoid unwanted pregnancies and STDs and succeed in not hurting each other or third parties and, most importantly, can in due course bring their children up in secure homes based

248

on mutual trust. But are not these good outcomes more *likely* down the other road?

There are many types and many different outlooks in this troubled world. This postscript was written so that you, reading this book, might know where I stand.

Glossary

abortion: loss of a pregnancy at any time before independent existence apart from the mother is deemed to be possible. Abortions may be *spontaneous* (= miscarriage) or *induced*, meaning caused to happen either legally or illegally. The general public often uses the word 'abortion' on its own to mean a legal induced abortion, but doctors prefer to use either that phrase or *termination of pregnancy*.

allergy: abnormal reactivity of an individual to a specific substance, following previous exposure to the same or a closely related substance. A similar process to *immunity* (below), but the *antibodies* produced are unwanted and can be harmful.

amine: an organic compound which contains nitrogen. The ones referred to in this book are present in the brain and believed to be important in its functions, both in health and disease.

anaemia: a decrease in the blood of the substance haemoglobin, carried by the red blood cells, which transports oxygen round the body.

androgenic: masculinizing.

antibodies: special substances produced by the body as a reaction to a foreign substance, or a substance which the body treats as foreign (page 208). Antibodies can be beneficial (as in *immunity*) or harmful (as in *allergy*).

'breakthrough' bleeding: any unexpected bleeding between hormone withdrawal bleeds ('periods') on the combined pill: i.e. bleeding on pill-taking days.

cervix: the narrow lower end of the *uterus*, containing the entrance to it. Sometimes called 'the neck of the womb'.

chloasma (= melasma): abnormal facial skin pigmentation occurring in some women during pregnancy or oral contraception.

chromosome: one of the microscopic thread-like structures visible in the nucleus of any body cell when it divides, carrying the genes. (Each gene controls the inheritance of a special characteristic of the individual – e.g. blood group or colour of the eyes.)

combined oral contraceptive: contraceptive which is taken by mouth and contains two hormones: one a *progestogen* and the other an *oestrogen.*

contraception: prevention of pregnancy by a reversible method. This definition excludes the other two types of birth control, which are sterilization and abortion. But see page 206.

contraceptive: any substance or device which produces contraception.

corpus luteum: the yellow body formed in the ovary during the menstrual cycle, arising from the largest follicle after it has discharged the egg.

cystitis: inflammation of the urinary bladder, usually caused by infection, causing a desire to pass urine more frequently and frequently a burning sensation on doing so.

D&C (Dilatation and Curettage): a very common minor operation in which the cervix is dilated, or enlarged sufficiently to allow a curette to be passed. This instrument is then used to scrape the lining on the inside of the uterus, in order to empty it, e.g. after a miscarriage or induced abortion which has been incomplete, or to obtain tissue for laboratory examination.

diabetes: strictly, should be *diabetes mellitus* – a disturbance of body chemistry causing an increase in the level of glucose in the blood after food, due to lack of the hormone insulin, or reduction in its effectiveness. These changes can lead to long-term complications, especially affecting the arteries.

ectopic pregnancy: a pregnancy in the wrong place – i.e. anywhere other than in the cavity of the uterus. The commonest site is in the uterine tube. It leads to the need for urgent operation, because the growing pregnancy can cause internal bleeding.

ejaculation: the spurting out of semen (sometimes called *the ejaculate*) from the end of the penis when a man has a climax.

embolism: transfer in the bloodstream of a mass, such as a blood clot from a vein, to lodge elsewhere, generally in the lungs (*pulmonary embolism*, page 79).

embryo: name given to the early pregnancy from the day of fertilization for about two months (then called the fetus).

endometrium: the special lining of the uterus, which is prepared by the hormones of the menstrual cycle in readiness for implantation of an embryo – or otherwise is shed at the menstrual period.

enzyme: a biological catalyst, which is a chemical which promotes the process of transformation of one substance to another within the body.

epididymis: a long tube coiled on itself to form a small linear structure attached to the testicle, and connecting it with the vas deferens.

ethinyloestradiol: one of the two artificial oestrogens which are used in combined oral contraceptive pills.

fertilization: the union of sperm and egg cell. The fertilized egg divides to produce an embryo and eventually a new individual.

fimbriae: the seaweed-like fronds which surround the outer end of each uterine tube, like a fringe.

follicle: a small fluid-filled balloon-like structure in the ovary, containing an egg cell. Only one, out of about twenty which enlarge in each menstrual cycle, normally releases a mature egg.

FSH (follicle stimulating hormone): the hormone, produced by the pituitary gland which stimulates the growth of follicles in the ovary; and hence causes the production of oestrogen and the maturing of an egg cell in the largest follicle.

hCG (human chorionic gonadotrophin): the hormone, produced by an early pregnancy, which travels to the ovary in the bloodstream and causes its corpus luteum to continue producing oestrogen and progesterone beyond its usual 14-day life span. The action of hCG is hence very similar to that of LH (see below).

hormone: a chemical substance produced in one organ and carried in the bloodstream like a 'chemical messenger' to another organ or tissue, whose function it influences or alters.

hypertension: high blood pressure, above the level which is accepted as normal (pages 86–7).

hysterectomy: an operation to remove the uterus.

immunity: resistance of the body to the effects of a foreign substance, resulting from the production of *antibodies* (see above) which are not harmful and often beneficial – unlike those produced as a result of *allergy*.

implantation: the process of embedding of the developing embryo in the endometrium.

IUD (intra-uterine device): a small plastic device, which may or may not also bear a chemical such as copper, which is inserted into the uterus to prevent pregnancy. Often called the 'coil' or 'loop'.

LH (luteinising hormone): the hormone produced by the pituitary gland which causes egg-release, and the production and maintenance of the corpus luteum.

libido: the internal urge or drive associated with the sexual instinct.

lipids: fats and associated chemical substances, carried in the blood.

mcg (microgram): this abbreviation is used for the metric unit which is one millionth of a gram in weight.

menopause: cessation of the menstrual periods due to failure of ovulation and hormone production by the ovaries. Often used inaccurately for the climacteric, the period of several years before and after periods actually cease.

menstrual cycle: the cycle of hormone and other changes in a woman's body which leads to a regular discharge of blood from the non-pregnant uterus.

mestranol: the less commonly used of the two artificial oestrogens which are used in combined oral contraceptive pills.

mucus: slippery fluid produced by mucous glands on the surface of a body structure. *Cervical mucus* is mucus produced by the glands of the cervix.

oestrogen: the female sex hormone produced by the ovary throughout the menstrual cycle. It is the hormone required to bring animals 'on heat', which occurs at the time called oestrus – hence the name oestrogen.

oestrogen-dominant pill: a combined pill whose biological effects on the body are due more to the relatively higher dose of oestrogen it contains than to the progestogen.

ovary: the female sex gland in which ova (egg cells) are developed and which is the main source of natural sex hormones.

ovulation: discharge of the ovum from the ovary – usually called egg-release in this book.

phlebitis: thrombosis and inflammation involving a vein – usually a superficial vein of the leg – which causes it to become hard and very tender.

pituitary gland: the gland, about the size of a pea, on a stalk at the base of the brain, which produces many important hormones including FSH and LH.

platelets: tiny particles circulating in the blood which are important in the early stages of thrombosis.

progesterone: the other main sex hormone produced by the ovaries (see *oestrogen*). This hormone is produced only in the second half of the menstrual cycle, by the corpus luteum. It prepares the body, especially the uterus, for pregnancy. It is one of the general class of *progestogens*. (A number of artificial progestogens are used along with an artificial oestrogen to produce the combined pill. Their names are given in Tables 8 and 9, pages 162, 163).

progestogen-dominant pill: a combined pill whose biological effects on the body are due more to the relatively higher dose of progestogen it contains than to the oestrogen.

prolactin: a hormone produced by the pituitary gland which stimulates the breasts to produce milk and is also involved in the menstrual cycle.

prostaglandins: natural substances manufactured and released within many tissues of the body. There are many different types with varying effects. Some natural prostaglandins cause the uterus to contract, and these and other artificial variants can therefore be used to cause an induced abortion.

puberty: the time when a boy or girl begins to develop secondary sex characteristics. In a girl, the most important event is the onset of periods, correctly called the menarche.

pyridoxine: this is another name for Vitamin B_6 and is important in body chemistry, particularly relating to the amines which have important functions in the brain.

RH (releasing hormone): there are in fact several releasing hormones, which travel down the stalk of the pituitary gland from the base of the brain, and cause it to release various hormones of its own into the bloodstream. In this book RH has been used to refer to the particular releasing hormone which makes the pituitary release LH and FSH.

spermicide: a substance which is capable of killing sperm. Recommended for contraception when used with another method such as the sheath or the cap, rather than used alone.

sterilization: an operation in a person of either sex which permanently prevents pregnancy, and which is either impossible or difficult to reverse. The definition therefore includes removal of the uterus, or of both ovaries or testicles, though these are only done when necessary because of some disease. More usually, sterilization is achieved by blocking a woman's uterine tubes or a man's vas deferens on each side.

subarachnoid haemorrhage: this is serious bleeding from a localized weakness of the wall of an artery in the brain, leading to blood appearing in the cerebro-spinal fluid which bathes the brain and spinal cord. It can be fatal or cause prolonged loss of consciousness, but recovery is possible, sometimes with the aid of surgery.

termination of pregnancy: see *abortion.*

testicle (testis): the sex gland of the male in which spermatozoa (sperm) develop, and which also manufactures male sex hormones, especially testosterone.

thrombosis: the formation of a blood clot within a blood-vessel (artery or vein).

uterus (womb): the hollow organ in women, like other mammals, in which the young develop during pregnancy.

uterine (Fallopian) tubes: the tubes which in the female convey the egg to the uterus, and in which fertilization by a sperm usually occurs.

vagina: the distensible passageway which extends from the cervix to the vulva, into which the penis is inserted during intercourse, and which also forms the main part of the birth canal during delivery of a baby.

vas deferens: the tube in the male which conveys the sperm from the epididymis to the base of the penis. It is the tube that is divided at *vasectomy.*

vulva: the name given to the female external genital structures.

100 woman-years: a measure of the frequency of an occurrence in this field. For example, a pregnancy rate of one per 100 woman-years for a given method means that one pregnancy can be expected among 100 women using it for one year (page 38).

Further reading

These and related titles are obtainable from the FPA Book Centre, Family Planning Association, 27–35 Mortimer Street, London WIN 7RJ (full book list available), or through a local bookshop if preferred. They should also be in most public libraries.

All titles are available in paperback editions unless otherwise stated.

A. Birth control – the methods

Belfield, T. and Martins, H. *Introduction to Family Planning,* Family Planning Association, 1984
   Brief, profusely illustrated booklet for the general public, written in simple language.
Hawkins, D. F. and Elder, M. G. *Human Fertility Control* Butterworth, 1979
   Comprehensive hardback textbook, with references, written primarily for doctors and medical students.
Kane, P. *The Which? Guide to Birth Control,* Consumers' Association, 1983.
   Helps the contraceptive user to make informed choices of methods and services.
Kleinman, R. L. *Family Planning Handbook for Doctors,* International Planned Parenthood Federation (IPPF), 1980.
   Readily understandable by anyone wanting a practical medical account of the available methods.
Potts, M. and Diggory, P. *Textbook of Contraceptive Practice,* Cambridge University Press, 1983.
   Presents a global view of all aspects of family planning, but emphasizing the common problems encountered in the West.
WOLS Committee *The Little Blue Book*, Oxford University Medical Society, 1983.
   By students for students – easily read information on all aspects of contraception and sexuality.

257

B. Induced abortion

Gardner, R. *Abortion – the Personal Dilemma,* The Paternoster Press, 1972.
   A unique, comprehensive account by a Christian gynaecologist of the medical, social, ethical, and spiritual issues of abortion. Also recommended: a cheap booklet by the same author and publisher, 1972, 'What about Abortion?'

Potts, M., Diggory, P., and Peel, J. *Abortion,* Cambridge University Press, 1977.
   A fascinating account of historical, sociological, clinical, and population aspects of abortion, worldwide.

Stirrat, G. M. 'Legalized Abortion – the Continuing Dilemma', Christian Medical Fellowship, 1979.
   Cheap and yet valuable booklet by a Christian gynaecologist, writing seven years after Gardner (see above).

C. Sexually transmitted diseases

Barlow, D. *Sexually Transmitted Diseases – The Facts*, Oxford University Press, 1981.
   Illustrated textbook, for a general readership. Dispels the fear and stigma attached to these common and readily treated conditions.

D. Sex and relationships

Delvin, D. *The Book of Love*, New English Library, 1983.
   Physical and emotional aspects of sex and marriage are explored together with helpful discussion of the problems.

Penrose, E. 'So Now You Know About Sex', British Medical Association, 1983.
   Cheap booklet for teenagers about growing-up, love, sex, and marriage.

Schaeffer, E. *What is a Family?*, Hodder and Stoughton, 1975.
   A personal view from one woman's experience.

Trobisch, W. *I Married You,* Inter-Varsity Press, 1972.
   An unusual, extremely readable book on marriage. Based on the author's experience in Africa, but relevant anywhere.

Warren, A. *Love Letters,* Scripture Union, 1979.
   Two people in love, a modern story told entirely by their own handwritten letters. True to life, challenging, sometimes painful – but ending on a note of hope.

E. Specially for women

Kilmartin, A. *Cystitis – The Complete Self-Help Guide,* Hamlyn (UK), Warner Books (USA), 1981.
Self-help for sufferers from common and often neglected problems. Discusses vaginal infections as well as cystitis.

Lanson, L. *From Woman to Woman,* Penguin, 1983.
Questions and answers about how a woman's body works and about gynaecological treatments.

Llewellyn-Jones, D. *Everywoman,* Faber, 1982.
A gynaecological guide for life, from puberty to the meno-pause.

Phillips, A. and Rakusen, J. *Our Bodies, Ourselves,* Penguin, 1983.
A health book by and for women. British edition of the original version by the Boston Women's Health Book Collective.

Stoppard, M. *Everywoman's Lifeguide,* Macdonald 1983.
How to achieve and maintain fitness, health and happiness in today's world.

F. History of birth control

Leathard, A. *The Fight for Family Planning,* Macmillan, 1980.
The history of the birth control movement in Britain from 1921. An uphill battle for recognition, culminating in 1974 in the agreement that family planning services should be provided within the National Health Service. Hardback.

Wood, C. and Suitters, B. *The Fight for Acceptance – a History of Contraception,* Medical and Technical Publishing, 1970.
The lessons of the past, starting at least 4,000 years ago – yet often still relevant today. Hardback.

G. World population, the environment, and related issues

McGraw, E. *Population Today,* Kaye and Ward, 1980.
An excellent, cheap, profusely illustrated readable book introducing world population and the related problems.

Medawar, J. *Lifeclass,* Hamish Hamilton, 1978.
Simply written and inexpensive illustrated hardback about the future. Human beings are the most gifted of the two million creatures who live on earth; by making right – or wrong – use of their powers, they alone can shape their own destiny.

Schumacher, E.F. *Small is Beautiful*, Sphere Books, 1974.
A study of economics as if people mattered.
Taylor, J. *Enough is Enough*, SCM Press, 1975.
A book by the Bishop of Winchester, condemning excess of all kinds and in favour of a simpler and more – not less – fulfilling life-style.
Ward, B. and Dubos, R. *Only One Earth*, Penguin, 1972.
Concerning the care and maintenance of a small planet.

H. Miscellaneous

Christopher, E. *Sexuality and Birth Control in Social and Community Work*, Maurice Temple Smith, 1980.
Information for the social and community worker about sexuality, contraception, abortion, and sexually transmitted diseases: the problems presented and how to cope with them.
Djerassi, C. *The Politics of Contraception*, W. H. Freeman, 1981.
Birth control in the year 2001 – critical issues and strategies for the future.
The King's Fund *The King's Fund Directory of Organisations for Patients and Disabled People*, King Edward's Hospital Fund for London. Distributed by Pitman Medical, 1979.
Pauncefort, Z. *Choices in Contraception*, Pan, 1984.
Choices, for men and for women.
Smith, M. and Kane, P. *The Pill off Prescription*, Birth Control Trust, 1975.
Reasons for widening the range of those empowered to dispense oral contraceptives.

Useful addresses

This list relates only to the British Isles and cannot be comprehensive. Only a few representative organizations are mentioned and details may have changed since this book went to press. If you have any difficulty, contact a similar-sounding organization, ask at your local Town Hall or Citizens' Advice Bureau, or telephone the Family Planning Association (FPA) (see below).

A. Birth control – and related matters

1. *Brook Advisory Centres*
   (Head Office)
   153A East Street
   London SE17 2SD   *Tel.* 01–708 1234

Centres providing a full service in birth control and related matters for young, usually unmarried people, without fuss and without fee.

2. *Family Planning Information Service*
   Family Planning Association
   27–35 Mortimer Street
   London WIN 7RJ   *Tel.* 01–636 7866

Perhaps the most useful address and telephone number of all. Gives free and confidential advice about all methods of birth control, sexual problems, clinics for sexually transmitted diseases (VD), and pregnancy testing. If you have an unplanned or unwanted pregnancy, it can help you to contact the organization of your choice for counselling and help – whether about abortion, adoption, or keeping the baby. Can also inform about other organizations, in this list and others not mentioned. A wide range of *free* leaflets available, about all aspects of sexuality.

3. *Irish Family Planning Association*
   Cathal Brugha Street Clinic
   Dublin 1   *Tel.* Dublin 727276 or 727363

Provides a similar service to the British FPA, but has to charge fees (according to how much you earn) and has to operate within the requirements of Irish law.

4. *Local Family Planning Clinics*

Addresses and opening times best obtained by looking under Family Planning in the yellow pages of your telephone directory. Otherwise contact 2 or 3 above.

5. *Margaret Pyke Centre for Study and Training in Family Planning*
   15 Bateman's Buildings
   Soho Square
   London WIV 5TW   *Tel.* 01–734 9351

The largest centre in Europe for free help with all aspects of birth control and fertility.

B. Counselling and more general advice

6. *British Association for Counselling*
   37A Sheep Street
   Rugby
   Warwickshire CV21 3BX   *Tel.* Rugby (0788) 78328

Provides an up-to-date list of local centres that can give expert help on problems concerning sex, drugs, accommodation, and many other matters.

7. *Care and Counsel*
   146 Queen Victoria Street
   London EC4

Counselling and psychotherapy from a Christian basis without strings and without moralizing. Please *write* for details or for an appointment.

8. *National Marriage Guidance Council*
   (Head Office)
   Herbert Gray College
   Little Church Street
   Rugby
   Warwickshire CV21 3AP   *Tel.* Rugby (0788) 73241

Has many local branches which run clinics for sexual, relationship, and marriage problems. Details from telephone directory or above.

9. *Rape Crisis Centre*
   PO Box 69
   London WC1X 9NJ   *Tel.* 01–837 1600 or 01–278 3956
Sympathetic and comprehensive advice about legal, medical, or any other matters, with moral support, for women who have been raped or sexually assaulted.

10. *Salvation Army Counselling Service*
    177 Whitechapel Road
    London E1 1DP   *Tel.* 01–247 0669
Counselling from a Christian basis without any strings or moralizing. Can also inform about help available locally if you live outside London. Also counselling in marital sexual dysfunction.

11. *The Samaritans*
    London: 39 Walbrook
    London EC4   *Tel.* 01–626 9000
Branches in most towns to help the lonely, despairing, or suicidal. Local numbers in the telephone directory.

C. Health

12. *Action on Smoking and Health (ASH)*
    5–11 Mortimer Street
    London W1N 7RJ   *Tel.* 01–637 9843
Everything to help the prospective ex-smoker.

13. *Health Education Council*
    78 New Oxford Street
    London WC1A 1AH   *Tel.* 01–637 1881
Information and free leaflets and posters on all aspects of how to stay healthy.

14. *Sexually Transmitted Diseases*
    Special Clinics
Local clinics are usually listed in the telephone directory under VD or Venereal Disease. Otherwise ask Casualty Department of local hospital or contact FPA (A2 above). There is also a comprehensive address list for the British Isles in the book by Barlow (see Further reading).

15. *Women's Health Concern*
    16 Seymour Street
    London W1H 5WB   *Tel.* 01–486 8653

Practical help with women's health problems, especially those related to the menstrual cycle and the menopause.

16. *Women's National Cancer Control Campaign*
    1 South Audley Street
    London W1Y 5DQ   *Tel.* 01–499 7532

Information and free leaflets on all aspects related to cancer in women.

D. People in special categories

NB The King's Fund, 126 Albert Street, London NW1 7NF (*Tel.*01–267 6111) publishes a book with numerous addresses of support groups for those with long-term illnesses of all kinds. See Further reading.

17. *Sexual and Personal Relationships of the Disabled (SPOD)*
    286 Camden Road
    London N7 0BJ   *Tel.* 01–607 8851

Help in a previously much-neglected area for people with any relevant disability.

E. Birth and babies, single parents

18. *Gingerbread*
    35 Wellington Street
    London WC2   *Tel.* 01–240 0953

A self-help group for one-parent families, with 300 branches.

19. *National Council for One-Parent Families*
    255 Kentish Town Road
    London NW5 2LX   *Tel.* 01–267 1361

Offers advice without strings or pressures, and in confidence. Acts as a link between self-help groups like 18, local social workers, and others providing services for single pregnant girls and single mothers or fathers.

20. *National Childbirth Trust*
    9 Queensborough Terrace
    London W2 3TB   *Tel.* 01–221 3833

Everything to help expectant mothers and fathers during pregnancy, childbirth, and breast-feeding. Issues leaflets and booklist, and address list for local classes (fees charged).

21. *Maternity Alliance*
    309 Kentish Town Road
    London NW5   *Tel.* 01–267 3255
Advises about getting fit for pregnancy. Send s.a.e. for leaflets.

F. World population, the environment, and related issues

A few of many organizations which might be mentioned. See pages 11–15 for further details about their work.

22. *Conservation Society*
    12A Guildford Street
    Chertsey
    Surrey KT16 9BQ   *Tel. Chertsey* (09328) 60975

23. *Friends of the Earth*
    377 City Road
    London EC1V 1NA   *Tel.* 01–837 0731

24. *International Planned Parenthood Federation*
    18–20 Lower Regent Street
    London SW1Y 4PW   *Tel.* 01–839 2911
(This links together the individual Family Planning Associations of the world.)

25. *Oxfam (Oxford Committee for Famine Relief)*
    274 Banbury Road
    Oxford OX2 7DZ   *Tel.* Oxford (0865) 56777

26. *Population Concern*
    231 Tottenham Court Road
    London W1   *Tel.* 01–631 1546 or 01–637 9582

27. *Tear Fund (The Evangelical Alliance Relief Fund)*
    11 Station Road
    Teddington
    Middlesex TW11 9AA   *Tel.* 01–977 9144

World directory of pill names

Only pills containing 50 mcg of oestrogen or less are listed, and all so-called 'sequential' pills are omitted. The directory is based on the *Directory of Contraceptives* published by the International Planned Parenthood Federation, 1981, in consultation with Philip Kestelman. The groups by letter A to F are those used in Table 8 (page 162), Table 9 (page 163), Table 11 (page 194), and Figure 15 (page 165), so that a pill brand identified here can be fitted into the scheme described in Chapters 7 and 8. *Caution*: Rarely, the same or a very similar name is used in different parts of the world for different formulations (e.g. Noriday). So recheck the stated formulation of a pill in the list here against that of any previously used packet which you are attempting to match, and discuss the matter with a doctor or pharmacist. He or she can also tell you if a 28-day (Every Day) version is available, if not mentioned here (see pages 42, 51).

Those pill brands which are available in Britain are in *italics*.

Abbreviations

Oestrogens		ethinyloestradiol	EE
		mestranol	MEE
Progestogens	Group A	levonorgestrel	LNG
	Group B	desogestrel	DSG
	Group C	norethisterone (in N. America called norethindrone)	NET
	Group D	norethisterone acetate (in N. America called norethindrone acetate)	NEA
	Group E	ethynodiol diacetate	EDDA
	Group F	lynestrenol	LYN
Miscellaneous (not used in Britain/USA)		chlormadinone acetate	CMA
		medroxyprogesterone acetate	MPA
		norgestrienone	NGT
		quingestanol acetate	QGA

$^+$means that the pill also contains (non-contraceptive) dextronorgestrel

Group A (Levonorgestrel, LNG)

Micrograms   Milligrams

EE 50 +	LNG 0.25	Anfertil,$^+$ Denoval, Euginon$^+$, Eugynon 0.25, Eugynon,$^+$ *Eugynon 50*,$^+$ Eugynona,$^+$ Evanor,$^+$ Evanor-d, Femenal,$^+$ Follinett, Follinyl,$^+$ Gentrol,$^+$ Mithuri,$^+$ Monovar, Neogentrol, Neogynona, Neogynon, Neo-Primovlar, Neovlar, Noral, Nordiol, Novogyn, Novogynon, Ovadon, Ovidon, Ovlar, Ovoplex, Ovral,$^+$ Ovral 0.25 mg, *Ovran*, Pil KB, Primovlar,$^+$ Promovlar 50,$^+$ Stediril,$^+$ Stediril-d.
EE 50 +	LNG 0.125	Ediwal, Gravistat 125, Microgynon, Microgynon 50, Minigynon 50, Minules, Neogentrol 125/50, Neo-Stediril, Regunon.
EE 30 +	LNG 0.25	*Eugynon 30, Ovran 30*, Primovlar 30.$^+$
EE 30 +	LNG 0.15	Egogyn, Follimin, Gynatrol, Lo-Ovral,$^+$ Microginon, Microgyn, *Microgynon 30*, Microvlar, Minidril, Minigynon 30, Minivlar, Min-Ovral,$^+$ Neogentrol 150/30, Neomonovar, Neovletta, Nordet, Nordette, Ovoplex 30/150, Ovoplexin, Ovral L,$^+$ Ovranet, *Ovranette*, Rigevidon, Stediril-d 150/30, Stediril-m.

Biphasic formulae

EE 50 +	LNG 0.05	Binordiol, Biphasil, Perikursal, Sequilar, Sequilarum, Sekvilar.
EE 50 +	LNG 0.125	
EE 30 +	LNG 0.15	Adépal.
EE 40 +	LNG 0.2	

Triphasic formula

EE 30 +	LNG 0.05	*Logynon, Logynon ED*, Triagynon, Trigynon, Trikvilar, *Trinordiol*, Triogyn, Trionetta, Triphasil, Triquilar, Triquilar ED. See page 162.
EE 40 +	LNG 0.075	
EE 30 +	LNG 0.125	

Group B (Desogestrel, DSG)

Micrograms   Milligrams

EE 30 +	DSG 0.15	*Marvelon*, Microdiol.

Biphasic and triphasic formulae
(To be announced).

Group C   (Norethisterone, NET)

Micrograms   Milligrams

EE 50 +	NET 1	Alovan, Arona, Ovcon 50.
MEE 50 +	NET 1	Anogenil, Conceplan, Conlumin, Floril, Gulaf, Maya, Nor-50, Noriday 1+50 Fe, *Norinyl-1*, *Norinyl-1/28*, Norinyl 1+50. Novulon 1/50, Orthonett, Orthonett 1/50, *Ortho-Novin 1/50*, Ortho-Novum 1/50, Perle, Plan mite, Regovar, Regovar 50, Ultra-Novulane.
EE 50 +	NET 0.4	Micropil.
EE 35 +	NET 1	Brevicon-1, Brevinor-1, Neocon, *Neocon 1/35*, *Norimin*, Norinyl 1+35, Norquest-Fe, Ortho-Novum 1/35, Ovysmen 1/35.
EE 35 +	NET 0.5	Brevicon, *Brevinor*, Conceplan mite, Moda Con, Modacon, Modicon, Norminest-Fe, Orthonett-Novum, *Ovysmen*, Ovysmen 0·5/35.
EE 35 +	NET 0.4	Ovcon 35, Oviprem.

Biphasic formulae

MEE 50 + NET 1 } MEE 50 + NET 2 }		Norbiogest.
EE 35 + NET 0.5 } EE 35 + NET 1 }		*Binovum*, Ortho-Novum 10/11 (equivalent to *Binovum*, page 162, but gives 3 extra days at the lower dose).

Triphasic formulae

EE 35 + NET 0·5 } EE 35 + NET 0.75 } EE 35 + NET 1 }	Ortho-Novum 7/7/7, *Trinovum*. See page 162.

Group D   (Norethisterone acetate, NEA)

Micrograms   Milligrams

EE 50 +	NEA 4	Anovial, *Anovlar 21*, Anovlar.
EE 50 +	NEA 3	Anovlar 3 mg, Anovlar mite, Ginovlar, Gyn-Anovlar, Gynovlar, *Gynovlar 21*, Profinix.
EE 50 +	NEA 2.5	Etalontin, *Norlestrin*, Norlestrin 2.5/50, Orlest 2.5, Prolestrin.
EE 50 +	NEA 2	Econ, Gynovlane.
EE 50 +	NEA 1	Anovlar 1 mg, Anovulatorio MK 1, Berligest, Celapil, Estrinor, Logest 1/50, Milli-Anovlar, *Minovlar, Minovlar ED*, Non-Ovlon, Norit, Norlestrin 1 mg, Norlestrin

1/50, Norlestrin Fe 1 mg, Orlest, *Orlest 21*, Orlest 1 mg, Prolestrin, Rosanil, Zorane 1/50.

EE 30 +	NEA 1.5	*Loestrin 30,* Loestrin 1.5/30, Loestrin Fe 1.5/30, Logest 1.5/30, Zorane 1.5/30.
EE 30 +	NEA 1	Econ 30, Loestrin 30, Trentovlane.
EE 30 +	NEA 0.6	Neorlest.
EE 20 +	NEA 1	*Loestrin 20,* Loestrin 1/20, Loestrin Fe 1/20, Minestrin 1/20, Nogest, Zorane 1/20.

Biphasic formulae

EE 50 +	NEA 1	Gynophase, Sinovular.
EE 50 +	NEA 2	
EE 30 +	NEA 1	Miniphase.
EE 40 +	NEA 2	

Group E   (Ethynodiol diacetate, EDDA)

Micrograms   Milligrams

EE 50 +	EDDA 1	Alfames E, Bisecurin, Demilen, Demulen, Evane, Gynorm, Hemovulen, Neovulen, Ovulen, Ovulen 1/50, *Ovulen 50,* Ovulène 50, Ovulen-Novum.
MEE 50 +	EDDA 1	Agestin, Angravid.
EE 50 +	EDDA 0.5	Anoryol, Demulen 50, Ovulen 0.5/50, Ovulen ½ 50.
EE 30 +	EDDA 2	*Conova 30,* Demulen 30.

Group F   (Lynestrenol, LYN)

Micrograms   Milligrams

EE 50 +	LYN 2.5	Anovulatorio, Lindiol, Lindiol 2.5, Lindión. Lyndiol, Lyndiol 2.5, Lyndiol neu, *Minilyn*, Neo-Lyndiol, Nonovulen, Noracyclin, Orgalutin, Ovariostat.
EE 50 +	LYN 1	Anacyclin, Lyndiol 1 mg, Lyndiolett, Microcyclin, Miniol, Ovoresta, Ovostat, Pregnon.
EE 40 +	LYN 2	Ermonil, Yermonil.
EE 37.5 +	LYN 0.75	Ginotex, Lyndiol 0.75, Micro-Ovostat, Minilyndiol, MiniPregnon, Ministat, Ovoresta M, Ovostat-Micro, Pregnon, Restovar.

Biphasic formula

EE 50 +	LYN 0.1	Fysioquens, Normophasic, Normophasico,
EE 50 +	LYN 1	Physiostat.

Miscellaneous – pills with progestogens not used in British Isles/USA

Micrograms	Milligrams	
MEE 50 +	CMA 2	Femigen.
EE 50 +	MPA 5	Nogest, Regulene.
EE 50 +	NGT 2	Planor.
EE 50 +	NGT 0.5	Miniplanor, Neo-Previson.
EE 50 +	QGA 0.5	Piloval, Reglovis, Relovis, Riglovis.

Continuous progestogen-only pills (POPs)

	Milligrams	
Group A	LNG 0.0375	*Neogest,*[+] Ovrette.[+]
	LNG 0.03	Follistrel, Microlut, Microluton, *Microval*, Mikro-30, *Norgeston*.
Group C	NET 0.35	Conceplan-Micro, Dianor, Micronett, *Micronor,* Micro-Novum, Micronovum, *Noriday,* Noridei, Nor-QD.
	NET 0.3	Conludag, Gesta Plan, Mini-Pe, Minipill.
Group D	NEA 0.6	Milligynon.
Group E	EDDA 0.5	Continuin, *Femulen*.
Group F	LYN 0.5	Exlutena, Exluton, Exlutona, Minette.
Miscellaneous	QGA 0.3	Demovis, Pilomin.

Stop-press

A new progestogen known as gestodene is under intensive study, in combination with ethinyloestradiol (EE). Fixed-dose and phased versions are expected to be marketed in 1985. Formulations and names to be announced.

Phased pills: for comparison with the others, the average daily doses given in the British brands are shown below:

	Micrograms	Micrograms
Logynon/Trinordiol	EE 32.4 +	LNG 92
Binovum	EE 35 +	NET 833
Trinovum	EE 35 +	NET 750

Index

For names of pills, see World directory of pill names (page 266) and Chapters 7, 8. Appendices (pages 229 onwards) are not indexed. See Glossary (page 250) for definitions of technical terms.

bones and joints, 115
bowel thrombosis, 85
brain
  as hormone controller, 24, 190, 195;
  see also pituitary gland; side-effects
  of pill on, 93–8; see also specific types
  of brain disease
breaks from pill-taking, 63, 104–10,
  126–30; between pill packets,
  effectiveness during, 43, 51–2, 57
breakthrough bleeding, 44, 46, 49, 53,
  57, 59, 60, 133, 169–70, 171, 172,
  174–6; and epilepsy, 98; when taking
  other drugs, 57, 58, 98, 159, 172
breast-feeding, 40; and the pill, 46,
  147, 184, 196, 225; contraceptive
  effect of, 15, 184, 210
breasts
  cancer, 114, 120–1, 153; check at
  family planning visit, 66; benign
  disease, 114, 121, 132, 138, 145, 170,
  178; enlargement, 113, 178; milky
  discharge, 72, 113–14;
  self-examination procedure, 66, 121,
  161; tenderness and tingling, 60, 114,
  170, 178, 192
breathlessness, 61
bursitis, 118

calf pain, 61, 79, 80; see also deep
  venous thrombosis
cancer
  and the pill, 119–24, 129–30; and
  smoking, 41, 91; past history of, 153;
  see also breast; cervix; ovary; uterus;
  vagina
candida infection, 103
cap, 2,18, 49, 88, 159, 205, 222, 224,
  225, 227
carpal tunnel syndrome, 62, 118
CASH Study, 120, 121, 122
central nervous system, 93–8
cerebral haemorrhage, 84
cerebral thrombosis, 83–4; see also
  strokes
cervix, 25, 36; cancer of, 21, 91, 122,
  153; cervical erosion, 102, 176;
  cervical mucus, 36, 38, 103, 104, 182,
  183, 184, 202; cervical ring, 203;
  cervical smear test, 21, 67, 69, 122,
  153, 161; trans-cervical sterilization,
  207
chest pain, 61
chicken pox, 118
chilblains, 118

Chinese Medical Journal, 216
chloasma, 115, 134, 139, 196
cholesterol, see blood fats
chorea, 98, 154
choriocarcinoma, 123
cilia, 27
circulatory disorders, 70–92, 126–9,
  130–3; family history of, 155–6; past
  history of, 149–52
clotting factors, 72, 77–8, 126, 130
coil, see IUD
collagen diseases, 152
combined pill
  compared with other methods, 220–4;
  contra-indications, 149–60, 194;
  duration of use, effect of, 88, 109–10,
  126–30, 158; history, 34–6; how it
  works, 30, 34, 36–41; ideal scheme
  for safe use, 160–1, 171–9; past use,
  possible effects of, 110–11, 126–30;
  rules for starting to take, 43–8, 65,
  169; see also specific diseases;
  side-effects of combined pill;
  Chapters 2–7, 10
conception, 27, 29; after coming off
  pill, 63, 109–10, 127, 187–90
condom, see sheath
cone biopsy, 153
contact lenses, 98
contraception
  future new methods, 200–19; history,
  8–11; ideal method, 197–8; present
  choices, 220–8; proportion using
  various methods in UK, 18; see also
  specific methods
contra-indications
  to combined pill, 149–60, 194; to
  POP, 192–3
coronary thrombosis, see heart disease
corpus luteum, 25, 26, 27, 28, 29, 32,
  33, 41; and other contraceptive
  methods, 205, 208–9; see also luteal
  phase; luteinising hormone
counselling, 1, 22–3, 65, 67–8, 69, 95–6,
  175
cramps
  menstrual, 33, 107, 138, 172; as
  affecting legs, 60, 118
Crohn's disease, 100, 118
cystitis, 101
cysts, ovarian, 106, 138, 192

D & C, 48, 123, 195
danazol, 215
deafness, 154

273